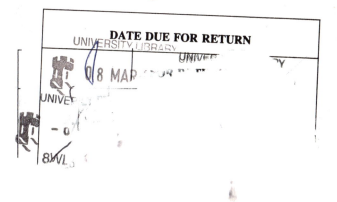

A History of Stroke

A History
of Stroke

Its Recognition and Treatment

William S. Fields, M.D.
Noreen A. Lemak, M.D.

Department of Neuro-Oncology
The University of Texas
M.D. Anderson Cancer Center
Houston, Texas

New York   Oxford
OXFORD UNIVERSITY PRESS
1989

Oxford University Press

Oxford   New York   Toronto
Delhi   Bombay   Calcutta   Madras   Karachi
Petaling Jaya   Singapore   Hong Kong   Tokyo
Nairobi   Dar es Salaam   Cape Town
Melbourne   Auckland

and associated companies in
Berlin   Ibadan

Copyright © 1989 by Oxford University Press, Inc.

Published by Oxford University Press, Inc.,
200 Madison Avenue, New York, New York 10016

Oxford is a registered trademark of Oxford University Press

Library of Congress Cataloging-in-Publication Data

Fields, William S. (William Straus), 1913–
   A history of stroke : its recognition and treatment / William S.
Fields and Noreen A. Lemak.
      p.   cm.
   Includes bibliographies and index.
   ISBN 0-19-505755-4
   1. Cerebrovascular disease—History.   I. Lemak, Noreen A.
II. Title.
   [DNLM: 1. Cerebrovascular Disorders—history.   WL 355 F463h]
RC388.5.F524 1989
616.8'1—dc 19
DNLM/DLC   88-23847
for Library of Congress   CIP

9 8 7 6 5 4 3 2 1
Printed in the United States of America

PREFACE

It is a tragedy that so many of us learn so little from history that could guide us now and in the future. Historians research, record, and attempt to interpret the past and the present in an endeavor to give us glimpses and sometimes whole accounts of what our forebears accomplished and what they failed to do or to recognize.

Even from our list of contents, the reader will see that much of contemporary understanding of cerebrovascular disease was gained in a remarkably brief period—perhaps no more than the span of our own lifetimes. Yet, as we became involved in this labor of love, writing about a scene that has been part of our life's work, we found that a great deal of the medical knowledge acquired in the recent past, with the help of sophisticated tools, had been understood deductively and previously described by those who had taken time to observe and record their findings.

This volume is filled with examples of how astute students of earlier days, who were able to evaluate their observations and then translate them into concepts, were prevented by technical limitations from putting them into practice. Only recently have the means come to hand for accurate detection, effective treatment, and prevention of circulatory disorders that may have a dramatic and often devastating effect on the brain and have been known to have serious consequences for the course of our world.

We are, of course, not so naive as to believe that the impact of what we decided to commit to print will be so profound that those who do follow us will not want to improve and add to the story.

To learn about the past, most students of medicine today rely almost exclusively on the computer files of the National Library of Medicine in Bethesda or similar files in other countries. Unfortunately, these files cover only a limited period in retrospect, and few students are interested in learning about accomplishments which antedate the creation of the files.

In reporting contemporary history, one always runs the risk of slighting someone by assigning credit or priority for discoveries incorrectly. Although we, ourselves, were participants in some of the events included, we tried to present this chronicle in an unbiased, objective, and dispassionate manner. We hope that we will be forgiven if we have overlooked anyone.

If we are able to give the reader some insight into past events that have had an influence on our treatment of strokes today and may lead to future progress, we judge our time and effort to have been spent well. We are grateful to colleagues in many medical disciplines who directed us to source material or provided clues from their own work, particularly the late Dr. Lawrence McHenry, a colleague and friend, whose pioneering work in the history of neurology gave impetus to our efforts to expand on what he had so ably begun.

We acknowledge the patience and tireless effort of Dorothy Darilek Butler, who typed our manuscript, and the assistance provided by the editorial staff of the Department of Scientific Publications of The University of Texas M.D. Anderson Cancer Center.

Houston, Texas   W. S. F.
July 1988   N. A. L.

CONTENTS

A History of Stroke

1

From the Greek Period to 1915

The word "carotid" is derived from the Greek *karos*, meaning "deep sleep," and it is the name the Greeks gave to the blood vessels leading to the brain. They recognized the importance of these great vessels in supplying blood to the brain and were also aware that any impediment to this flow resulted in unconsciousness.

Hippocrates, about 400 B.C., observed that many blood vessels connect to the brain; some are slender, but two are stout. He believed that the arteries were filled with air, an idea gained from their emptiness in dead animals.[1] In his aphorisms on apoplexy many modern concepts are expressed, such as "Persons are most subject to apoplexy between the ages of 40 and 60," and "Unaccustomed attacks of numbness and anesthesia are signs of impending apoplexy."[2] A probable subarachnoid hemorrhage is also depicted:

> When persons in good health are suddenly seized with pains in the head, and straightway are laid down speechless, and breathe with stertor, they die in seven days, unless fever comes on.[2]

The *Epidemics* by Hippocrates describes puerperal hemiplegia and convulsions with paralysis of the right arm and loss of speech in what is probably the first written account of aphasia:

> A woman who lived on the sea-front was seized with a fever while in the third month of pregnancy. She was immediately seized with pains in the loins. On the third day, pain in the head, neck, and around the right clavicle. Very shortly the tongue became unable to articulate and the right arm was paralyzed following a convulsion. . . . Her speech was delirious. . . . Fourth day: speech was indistinct . . . reached a crisis and the fever left her.[1]

3

In the third century B.C., the modern idea of basing medicine on anatomy and physiology flourished in Alexandria, Egypt. Anatomy rooms were established for the dissection of bodies and it is claimed that Herophilus (300 B.C.) dissected hundreds. He is also given credit for stating that the pulse does not result from a mysterious power within the arteries themselves but that this power is communicated to them by the action of the heart—the systole and diastole. Herophilus described the ventricles and venous sinuses of the brain, particularly the confluence of the sinuses (torcular Herophili). He was the first to formulate the concept of the "rete mirabile" (Figure 1.1)—a vascular plexus or network of blood vessels at the base of the brain surrounding the pituitary gland. This concept was given support by the dissections performed by Galen (A.D. 131–201), and in the sixteenth century Vesalius made drawings of the rete mirabile.

The most complete account of Roman medicine is that of Aurelius Celsus (25 B.C.–A.D. 50), who described "apoplexy" and differentiated it from "paralysis" by noting that in the former the whole body is paralyzed, while the effects of the latter are localized. Aretaeus of Cappadocia also wrote of apoplexy as a paralysis of the entire body including sensation, understanding, and movement. He pointed out that paralysis is on the side of the body opposite the affected side of the head due to crossing of the nervous pathways:

> If, therefore, the commencement of the affection be below the head, such as the membrane of the spinal marrow, the parts which are homonymous and connected with it are paralyzed: the right on the right side, the left on the left side. But if the head be primarily affected on the right side, the left side of the body will be paralyzed; and the right, if on the left side.[1,3]

From this quotation it seems that Aretaeus was aware of the information gained from Galen's experiments on the spinal cord. He expanded the description of crossed function beyond what was noted by Galen. In reasoning why paralysis occurs on the side opposite the lesion, Artaeus wrote:

> The cause of this is the interchange in the origin of nerves, for they do not pass along on the same side, the right on the right side, until their termination; but each of them passes over to the other side from that of its origin, decussating each other in the form of the letter X.[1,3]

Galen followed Hippocrates in attributing apoplexy to an accumulation of phlegm in the arteries of the brain that obstructed the passage of animal spirits from the ventricles. Hippocrates had spoken of severe and mild forms of apoplexy, but Galen divided the condition into four varieties

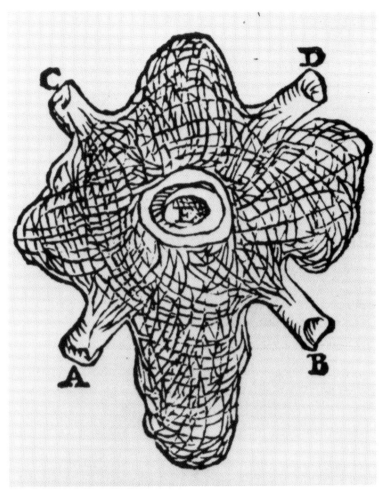

Figure 1.1. Drawing by Vesalius showing the ancient concept of the rete mirabile, which was first described by Herophilus and later given further support by Galen's dissections. The rete mirabile is a vascular plexus or network of blood vessels at the base of the brain surrounding the pituitary gland, E. This vascular formation occurs in lower mammals, but not in man. A and B are the arteries "that run below the skull" and C and D indicate the vessels coming from the plexus. The fact that the rete appeared in the early illustrations of the brain suggests that most of the dissections must have been of animals rather than of man. (From Garrison FH: *History of Neurology.* Revised and enlarged by McHenry LC, Jr., 1969. Courtesy of Charles C Thomas, Publisher, Springfield, IL)

according to the degree that respiration was affected. An apoplectic was generally one who became suddenly senseless as if struck by lightning, with loss of all motion except that of respiration. The predisposing causes were considered to be emotion, plethora, sloth, drunkenness, and gluttony. Galen, Hippocrates, and Aretaeus agreed that the worst forms of apoplexy were those in which stertor and foaming at the mouth occurred. Galen correctly attributed death in such cases to failure of respiration. Much later Caelius Aurelianus (A.D. fifth century) pointed out the occurrence of apoplexy accompanied by scintillation scotoma–implying an association between migraine and apoplexy.[1,4] Paul of Aegina (A.D. 625–690) seems to have been the first to use the term "hemiplegia," which is not found in earlier writings, although the condition was well known.[1]

The erroneous notion of the rete mirabile as described by Herophilus and later by Galen was denied by Jacopo Berengario da Carpi (c. 1470–1550), who stated that it did not exist in human beings.[1]

Andreas Vesalius (1514–1564) propelled knowledge of the anatomy of the brain forward with one great bound since he was the first anatomist to rely on a sound foundation of observation for his studies (Figure 1.2).[5] Fortunately, the illustrations of Vesalius' dissections were rendered with remarkable clarity by an extraordinary artist, Jan Stephan Kalkar, and were reproduced both as woodcuts and copper plates. The seventh book of his *Fabrica* contains 15 diagrams of the brain, which are among the most outstanding neuroanatomical drawings ever produced.[6] The first dissection, representing a head from which the calvarium has been removed, accurately depicts the middle meningeal artery meandering across the surface of the dura. In general, Vesalius' description of the blood vessels is adequate, but he overlooked the hexagonal ring of communicating vessels at the base of the brain. Like da Carpi, he disputed Galen on the existence of the rete mirabile, stating that it is almost nonexistent in humans.

The leading neuroanatomist of the seventeenth century was Thomas Willis (1621–1675), who contributed the term "neurology" to medicine. Willis took the root "neuro" from the Greek word meaning "sinew," "tendon," or "bowstring"; the word "neurology" first appeared in Greek in his *Cerebri Anatome*.[7] Although Willis made many significant contributions to neurology and clinical medicine, the structure for which he is eponymously remembered was actually described by several others before him.[8,9] The arterial circle of vessels at the base of the brain was first mentioned as such in 1561 by Gabriel Fallopius (1523–1562).[1] He described the union and later the division of the vertebral arteries and the union of the anterior rami (corresponding to our anterior communicating arteries) to the carotid arteries. Only part of the posterior communicating

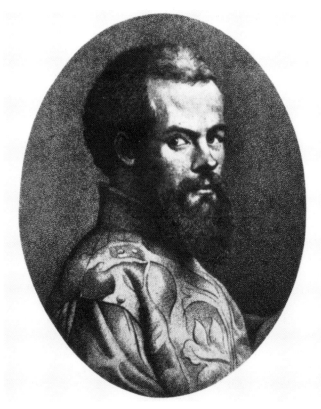

Figure 1.2. ANDREAS VESALIUS
(An engraving by T. Medland of a portrait by Titian)

artery was mentioned, and it had only an indirect connection with the external branch (corresponding to our middle cerebral artery) of the carotid artery. Fallopius' description resembles one side of the arterial circle shown in a drawing by Giulio Casserio (1545–1605), a professor at Padua and one of William Harvey's teachers. Casserio provided the first illustration of the circle of Willis, showing the complete union of the posterior communicating artery only on one side, perhaps a consequence of the frequent morphologic variations of these blood vessels.[1.10] The circle next appeared in the anatomical works of Johann Vesling (1595–1649), a professor of anatomy and surgery at Padua. In Vesling's plate the posterior cerebral arteries are absent, and the basilar artery divides into two large posterior communicating arteries.[1.11] Following Vesling's studies, another

Thomas Willis
described the
cycle of Willis

complete description of the circle and its anastomotic function was furnished by Johann Jakob Wepfer (1658)[12].

It seems reasonable to assume that these discrepancies in descriptions
of the arteries at the base of the brain can be ascribed to the frequency
with which congenital morphologic variants occur. In view of the fact
that such variants can be found in more than 60% of brains examined at
autopsy, it is not surprising that these earlier anatomists failed to recognize the complete "circle," which in most languages other than English
is referred to as a "polygon."[13]

Willis did not, in fact, claim sole credit for the description of the circle;
he acknowledged previous anatomical studies. Along with Wepfer, however, he was the first to recognize the clinical importance of the circle.
Willis records the clinical histories of two patients in whom he suggests
that this anatomical configuration prevented apoplexy or paralysis. One
of these patients had occlusions of both the right carotid and the right
vertebral arteries, but did not succumb to apoplexy during life. Willis
reasoned that the remaining large vessels flowing toward the arterial circle
at the base of the brain were able, by way of their "mutual conjoinings,"
to "supply or fill the channels and passages of all the rest."[1,7]

One of the most imaginative physiologists of the seventeenth century
was Willis' colleague at Oxford, Richard Lower (1631–1691), a pioneer
experimentalist whose scientific achievements were second only to those
of William Harvey. Lower's discovery that the blood changes its color
by deriving some "quality" when passing through the lungs was a landmark in the history of medicine. An associate of Willis for ten years,
Lower demonstrated the sufficiency of the arterial circle at the base of
the brain to maintain the cerebral circulation even when three of the four
arteries supplying the brain had been tied off.[1]

Significant advances in the understanding of brain pathology came with
studies of apoplexy. The earliest of these studies was performed by Gre-
gor Nymman (1594–1638) of Wittenberg, who published the first monograph on apoplexy in 1619.[1,14] Although his hypothesis of the cause of
apoplexy is intertwined with the erroneous theory of the movement of
vital spirits, Nymman did recognize that an apoplectic attack would occur
with the closure of the vessels or passageways that bore the vital spirits
to the brain. The most important progress in the investigation of apoplexy
came from the precise studies by the brilliant Johann Jakob Wepfer (1620–
1695) of Schaffhausen.[8,15,16] He performed meticulous examinations of
the cerebral blood vessels and the brains of patients who had had apoplexy. He dissected and traced the carotid and vertebral arteries from their
origins to their formation of the arterial circle at the base of the brain.

He was the first anatomist to illustrate the siphon of the carotid artery and to provide a clear description of the course of each cerebral artery including that of the middle cerebral in the Sylvian fissure.

That apoplexy often resulted from cerebral hemorrhage was little known before the publicaton of Wepfer's treatise on apoplexy (1658) (Figure 1.3), which was reprinted in five editions (the last in 1724).[1,12] He described four cases of cerebral hemorrhage varying from subarachnoid bleeding at the base of the brain to massive intracerebral hemorrhage. Wepfer accepted Harvey's concept of a closed loop of blood flow through the body, recognizing inflow through the carotid and vertebral arteries

Figure 1.3. JOHANN JACOB WEPFER
(From Garrison FH: *History of Neurology.* Revised and enlarged by McHenry LC, Jr., 1969. Courtesy of Charles C Thomas, Publisher, Springfield, IL)

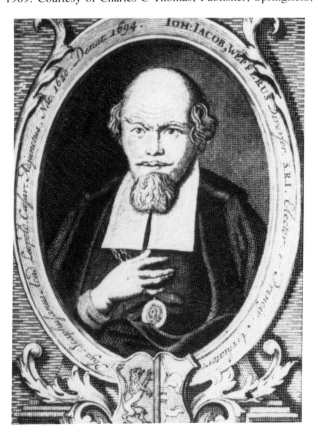

and discharge by way of the dural sinuses and jugular veins. He postulated that anything capable of obstructing the influx of blood to the brain and its return through the jugular veins was capable of producing apoplexy. He understood that extrinsic compression of the internal carotid or vertebral arteries or occlusion or narrowing of the lumen by corpora fibrosa (small fibrous bodies) in the vascular wall would impede a sufficient supply of blood from reaching the brain.[1]

Wepfer stated that those at greatest risk for apoplexy are the obese, those whose face and hands are livid, and those whose pulse is consistently irregular. This is the first implication that persons with hypertension or heart disease are more liable to suffer an apoplectic attack. Wepfer recognized that the clinical patterns of apoplexy are variable, and that the brain cannot survive deprivation of its nourishment for even a brief period of time. He also observed that some patients are immediately rendered unconscious, while others recover from an attack in a relatively short time and still others suffer a hemiplegia if only one side of the brain is involved. The character of the attack, in his opinion, depended on the amount and degree of arterial obstruction.[1]

Although Wepfer was the first to appreciate that apoplexy often resulted from cerebral hemorrhage, he was not definite in his opinion that the brain abnormality was on the side opposite the affected limbs. In most cases Wepfer expected to find the lesion on the same side. The actual demonstration of the mechanism of paralysis on the side opposite from the brain lesion in apoplexy was made by Domencio Mistichelli (1675–1715), a professor of medicine at the University of Pisa.[1,17] In his treatise on apoplexy, Mistichelli accepts the crossed relationship as a well-recognized fact but proceeds to provide details of his view of the anatomy of the brainstem by illustrating the decussation of the pyramids.[1,18] Despite the fact that his neuroanatomical examination was inaccurate, his concept of a pyramidal decussation was a new one. The illustration in his book shows a hemiplegic posture with outward rotation of the affected left limb. Mistichelli even went so far as to suggest that application of a hot cautery to the foot would cure the paralysis.[1]

Atherosclerosis of arteries had been observed by about 1500, but Francois Bayle (1622–1709) was among the first to relate it to apoplexy. Bayle described both calcification and plaques within the cerebral arteries.[1,19]

A firm basis for the study of pathology of the nervous system was established in the eighteenth century by Giovanni Battista Morgagni (1682–1771), a professor at the University of Padua.[1,20] Morgagni amassed a collection of case material over many years, and eventually published his classic *De Sedibus* at the age of 79 years.[21] This monumental work consisted of five volumes in which Morgagni recorded the postmortem findings together with the clinical case notes. This was the first time that such comprehensive material had been collected.

The first volume, *Of Disorders of the Head,* consisting of fourteen chapters, is probably the earliest work on neuropathology. The first chapter describes cases of pain in the head. The next four deal with apoplexy, which Morgagni divided into three categories—serous apoplexy, sanguinous apoplexy and apoplexy that is neither serous nor sanguinous. It is in these chapters that Morgagni first presents the evidence that the pathological lesion in apoplexy is on the side opposite the paralysis. This observation served to substantiate the theories of other observers back to at least Aretaeus.[1]

According to di Giacomo, Morgagni may have provided the first descripton of "pulseless disease."[22] A 40-year-old woman had been a patient on numerous occasions at his hospital during a period of six years. Her "radial pulse was never perceived." After her death from asthma, Morgagni had an opportunity to examine the body and describe how the aorta above the valves became "thicker and harder, while its internal layers, which in many places had become yellow, showed many signs of change into bone tissue, as could be noted at the outset of one of the subclavians."[21]

The English pathologist Matthew Baillie (1761–1823) in the final chapter of his *Morbid Anatomy* describes the "Diseased Appearances of the Brain and Its Membranes." In the part concerned with cerebral hemorrhage he writes:

> It is very common in examining the brain of persons who are considerably advanced in life, to find the trunks of the internal carotid artery upon the side of the sella turcica very much diseased, and this disease extends frequently more or less into the small branches. The disease consists in a bony or earthy matter being deposited in the coats of the arteries, by which they lose a part of their contractile and distentile powers, as well as of their tenacity. The same sort of diseased structure is likewise found in the basilar and its branches.

> The vessels of the brain, under such circumstances of disease, are much more liable to be ruptured than in a healthy state. Whenever blood is accumulated in unusual quantity, or the circulation is going on in them with unusual vigour, they are liable to this accident, and accordingly in either of these states ruptures frequently happen. Were the internal carotid arteries and the basilar artery not subject to the diseased alteration of structure

which we have described, effusions of blood within the cavity of the cranium, where there has been no previous external injury, would be very rare.[1,23]

In this manner Baillie directed attention to the fact that cerebral hemorrhage was the result of disease of the blood vessels of the brain, but he failed to recognize that vascular disease was also a cause of cerebral infarction.[1]

William Heberden (1710–1801), a highly regarded practitioner in London, described the manifestations of transient cerebral vascular insufficiency, which so often precede total paralysis:

> A faltering and inarticulation of the voice, drowsiness, forgetfulness, a slight delirium, a dimness of sight, or objects appearing double, trembling, a numbness gradually propagated to the head, a frequent yawning, weakness, a distortion of the mouth, a palpitation, a disposition to faint; some, or most of these have preceded a palsy for a few minutes, or for some hours, or even for a few days; and a weakness of a limb, or of one side, has been many months, or a few years, gradually increasing to a perfect loss of one side, or a hemiplegia. I have known a sleepiness and duplicity of objects with violent pains and tightness of the head for two days, then the senses and voice were lost and on the third the man expired. A numbness of the hand has come on the first day, on the second a faltering of the voice, and a palsy on the third.[1,24]

John Hunter was among the first to study collateral blood flow (Figure 1.4).[25] In 1785, after ligating the main artery to the rapidly growing antler of a stag, he noted no cessation of growth and observed the rapid appearance of enlarged superficial vessels that carried blood around the obstruction. He explained this phenomenon on the principle that "the blood goes where it is needed."[13] In treating a patient who had a popliteal aneurysm, Hunter applied his experiment by ligating the femoral artery (1786). The limb remained viable.[13,26]

One of the most remarkable contributions to eighteenth-century clinical neurology was the description of an affliction suffered by Gaspard Vieusseux,[27] a Swiss physician, who experienced what conforms in many respects to a lateral medullary syndrome of the brainstem. The signs and symptoms were most likely the result of occlusion of the posterior inferior cerebellar or the vertebral artery. Vieusseux himself recorded his experience and presented these observations to the Medical and Chirurgical Society of London on December 18, 1810. He reported severe discomfort with loss of pain sensation in the left half of his face and left facial paralysis, accompanied by vertigo, vomiting, dysarthria, dysphagia, ptosis

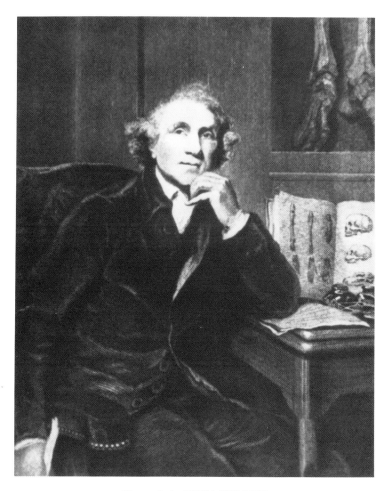

Figure 1.4. JOHN HUNTER
(An engraving by G. Adcock of a painting by Sir Joshua Reynolds)

of the left eyelid, and absence of sweating on the left half of his face. On the right side of his trunk he noted loss of pain and temperature appreciation and that his left extremities were weak. After recovering from the acute episode, he functioned well for more than five years until he was suddenly overcome by severe weakness of the left limbs, along with giddiness and weakness of the mouth and tongue. This case report of a medullary syndrome was recorded 85 years prior to the classic description by Wallenberg.[1,27]

The medical works of the Swedish botanist Carolus Linnaeus (1707–1778) include a description of aphasia that is probably the first to characterize the classical symptom of knowing what one wishes to say without being able to say it.[1,28] The patient portrayed by Linnaeus could comprehend both written and spoken language, but could not utter a word.[29] Among the most explicit descriptions of aphasia is that of von Swieten (1754) in his commentaries on the neurological observations of Hermann Boerhaave (1668–1738), the founder of Dutch medicine:

> I have seen many patients whose cerebral functions were quite sound after recovery from apoplexy, except for this one deficit: In designating objects, they could not find the correct names for them. These unfortunate people would try with their hands and feet and an effort of their whole body to explain what they wanted and yet could not. This disability remained incurable for many years.[1,30]

Another classical description of aphasia appears in the letters of Samuel Johnson (1709–1784):

> About three in the morning . . . I wakened . . . and sat up. . . . I felt a confusion and indistinctness in my head which lasted, I suppose, about half a minute. . . . Soon after I perceived that I had suffered a paralytic stroke and that my speech was taken from me. . . . My organs were so obstructed that I could say "No," but scarcely say "Yes". . . . I had no pain. . . . I put myself into violent motion. . . . But all was in vain. . . . I then wrote to Mr. Allen. . . . In penning this note I had some difficulty, my hand, I knew not how or why, made wrong letters. . . . Dr. Heberden and Dr. Brocklesby were called. . . . They put a blister upon my back, and two from my ear to my throat . . . before night I began to speak with some freedom, which has been increasing ever since.[1]

Garrison relates:

> In the chapter "Of Derangement of the Memory" in his classic psychiatry text, *Diseases of the Mind,* Benjamin Rush (1812) describes several types of aphasia as disturbances in memory. He mentions that patients may forget names or "vocables of all kinds." Others, forgetting names, may substitute a word in no way related. He recognized that multilingual patients may revert to another language when the facility for using one language is disturbed. Rush knew that Dr. Johnson forgot the words of the Lord's Prayer in English but attempted to repeat them in Latin.[1]

John Cheyne (1777–1836), better known for his description of periodic breathing (Cheyne-Stokes respiration), also wrote a classic treatise on apoplexy.[31] This treatise delineated Cheyne's concept of the role played by cerebral circulation in apoplexy. His work included the earliest illustration of a subarachnoid hemorrhage and also examples of cerebral infarction.[1] However, the first separate text on neurology may be that of John Cooke (1756–1838), a physician to the London Hospital (Figure 1.5). *A Treatise on Nervous Disease* (1820–1823) was compiled "after an experience in medicine of many years" and after a thorough search of the literature. The work is divided into three parts. The first volume, *On Apoplexy*, was presented in 1819 as the Croonian lecture (Figure 1.6).[32] Cooke's work includes in a lengthy introduction the first history of neurological thought from the ancients to the turn of the nineteenth century. It is so comprehensive that it has been recognized as the most important single contribution to neurology for its time.[1]

Figure 1.5. JOHN COOKE
(Courtesy of the Royal Society of Medicine, London)

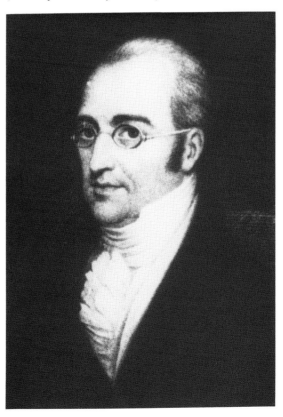

A

TREATISE

ON

NERVOUS DISEASES.

By JOHN COOKE, M.D. F.A.S.

FELLOW OF THE ROYAL COLLEGE OF PHYSICIANS, AND LATE PHYSICIAN
TO THE LONDON HOSPITAL.

IN TWO VOLUMES.

VOL. I.

ON APOPLEXY,

INCLUDING

APOPLEXIA HYDROCEPHALICA,

OR

WATER IN THE HEAD;

WITH AN

INTRODUCTORY ACCOUNT OF THE OPINIONS OF
ANCIENT AND MODERN PHYSIOLOGISTS,

RESPECTING THE

NATURE AND USES OF THE NERVOUS SYSTEM.

*Read at the College, as the Croonian Lectures of the
Year 1819.*

LONDON:

PRINTED FOR LONGMAN, HURST, REES, ORME, AND BROWN,
PATERNOSTER-ROW.

1820.

Figure 1.6. Title page of John Cooke's *Treatise on Nervous Diseases.* (From Garrison FH: *History of Neurology.* Revised and enlarged by McHenry LC. Jr., 1969. Courtesy of Charles C Thomas, Publisher, Springfield, IL)

The relationship of "softening of the brain" (infarction) to disease of the arteries may have been first clearly recognized in 1823 by Léon Rostan (1790–1866), a professor of medicine, lecturer, and writer in Paris.[33,34] Soon thereafter (1828), John Abercrombie also wrote of this association.[1,35] Sir Robert Carswell in his atlas of general pathology (1838) included 2000 watercolor drawings of diseased structures.[36] His examples of atherosclerosis of the cerebral arteries were particularly noteworthy.[1] Virchow, in Volume I of his *Archives*, was the first to point out that embolism is frequently a cause of brain softening.[37]

According to Robicsek, the earliest report of operative ligation of the common carotid artery was that of Ambrose Paré, the French court physician, in 1552.[38] His patient, unfortunately, became aphasic and hemiplegic. Elective ligation of the common carotid artery with symptom-free survival was performed by Hebenstreit and reported in 1793.[38]

In 1803, Fleming, a naval surgeon, ligated the common carotid artery in a young man on board ship who had attempted suicide by cutting his own throat. Testimony to the operation was given by an assistant surgeon who wrote a statement headed "Case of Rupture of the Carotid Artery, and Wounds of Several of Its Branches, successfully treated by tying the common Trunk of the Carotid itself."[39]

Cooper (1836) described his observations following ligation of the principal cervical arteries in a dog, accompanied by interruption of the vagus, phrenic, and sympathetic nerves.[40] He was impressed by the fact that the function of the brain was not altered as far as he could determine. Chevers (1845)[41] published the earliest comprehensive review of the consequences of obliteration of the carotid arteries on the cerebral circulation.[1]

Robicsek relates:

> In 1839, John Davy reported a case of a 55-year-old army officer with absent arterial pulses in his arms who had symptoms of cerebrovascular insufficiency. . . . The patient died from a ruptured syphilitic aneurysm of the aorta, which turned out to be the cause of obstruction of the arch branches.[38,42]

Ellis (1845) reported the astonishing experience of successful ligation of both carotid arteries in a 21-year-old patient who sustained a gunshot wound of the neck and tongue when he was mistaken for a bear by a companion. This occurred while he was setting a trap in the woods near Grand Rapids, Michigan, on October 21, 1844. Approximately one week later Ellis had to ligate the patient's left carotid artery because of hemorrhage from the tongue wound. An appreciation of the surgeon's problem can be gained from Ellis' description of the operation:

> We placed him on a table. . . . I ligatured the left carotid artery, below the omohyoideus muscle; an operation attended with a good deal of difficulty, owing to the swollen state of the parts, the necessity of keeping up pressure, the bad position of the parts owing to the necessity of keeping

the mouth in a certain position to prevent his being strangulated by the blood, and the necessity of operating by candle light.[43]

There was recurrent hemorrhage on the eleventh day after the accident and right carotid artery pressure helped control the blood loss. Therefore, it was necessary to ligate the right carotid artery as well four and one-half days after the left carotid artery had been ligated. Ellis remarked:

> For convenience we had him in the sitting position during the operation; when we tightened the ligature, no disagreeable effects followed; no fainting, no bad feeling about the head; and all the perceptible change was a slight paleness, a cessation of pulsation in both temporal arteries, and of the hemorrhage.[43]

The patient recovered rapidly with good wound healing and returned to normal daily activity. There was no perceptible pulsation in either superficial temporal artery.[44]

The fact that alterations in the cerebral circulation might be related to "cerebral accidents" or apoplexy was brought out in the clinical and experimental studies of Burrows (1846), who accumulated considerable evidence to support the idea of a relationship between cerebral anemia and apoplexy.[1,45] He was the first to indicate that the effects of cerebral anemia could be produced not only by obvious anemia itself, but also from a fall in blood pressure to a level where it was insufficient to supply blood to the brain. Burrows also observed that cardiac and apoplectic symptoms may occur simultaneously. He carried out some of the earliest studies of the physiology of the cerebral circulation and, in his Lumleian Lecture of 1843–1844, reported that the amount of blood in the brain can vary, and that this variation might be responsible for clinical signs. Burrows' work was a milestone in the study of cerebral vascular physiology.

Although some authors credit Durand-Fardel (1843)[46] with the first description of cerebral lacunes, it was found that the term "lacune" was used first by Dechambre in 1838.[47] At that time, apoplexy was still considered a uniformly fatal disease, but Dechambre, then an intern at the Hôpital de la Salpêtrière in Paris, observed several patients who survived and improved after a stroke and then showed lacunes at autopsy. On May 19, 1838, Dechambre published a "Memoir on the Curabilility of Cerebral Softening."[48] His case 9, a patient who had recovered from acute hemiplegia, disclosed the following on postmortem examination:

> . . . a number of small lacunes, of variable size and form, more or less filled with a milky fluid . . . resulting from liquefaction and partial reabsorption in the center of the (cerebral) softening. According to the degree

of hardening and reabsorption of the liquified (cerebral) pulp these lacunes appear empty or stay more or less filled. . . . It is, no doubt, with small foci of partial softening, that these round cavities without membranes should be correlated.[49]

William W. Gull wrote of a "Case of Occlusion of the Innominate and Left Carotid" in 1855,[50] but William Scovell Savory's "Case of a Young Woman in Whom the Main Arteries of Both Upper Extremities and of the Left Side of the Neck were Throughout Completely Obliterated" is considered to be a landmark article on cerebral ischemia.[51] Savory presented a detailed case history and postmortem findings of a 22-year-old woman who had no perceptible pulse in any of the vessels of the head, neck, or upper extremities; the femorals and the vessels of the lower extremities pulsated weakly; a bruit could be detected over the right common carotid. She had multiple complaints over several years: weakness, dizziness, seizures, limb paralysis, pain in the head, and ulceration of the scalp which destroyed bone and extended into the cerebral hemisphere. At autopsy, "all the main arteries of both upper extremities and of the left side of the neck were reduced to solid cords, and presented the exact condition of vessels through which the flow of blood had been for some time mechanically arrested." He believed that the changes in the arteries were the result of inflammation, with the inner coat having undergone the most extensive alteration. This differed from the opinion of Rokitansky on the pathology of arteritis. In his *Pathologische Anatomie*, Rokitansky wrote that "the absence of vessels in the circular fibrous coat, and more especially in the inner coat of the vessels, forbids our assuming the possibility of inflammation in these layers."[51] Savory wrote, "There can be no doubt concerning the origin of the fibrous cord which filled up the interior of the contracted vessels. It was evidently the remains of the blood which had coagulated in the canal, and which had undergone changes similar to those that occur in the clot which forms in an artery beyond the point where a ligature has been applied."[51]

Gurdjian and Gurdjian state:

In the latter part of the Nineteenth Century, carotid occlusive disease in the neck was recognized clinically because of a combination of visual disturbance (blindness or amaurosis fugax) and focal paralytic involvement. In 1856, Virchow[53] described carotid thrombosis with ipsilateral blindness. However, he found the lumina of the ophthalmic and central retinal arteries to be patent.[52]

Kussmaul (1872) described a carotid artery thrombosis in the neck accompanied by visual disturbance of the homolateral eye.[52,54]

Gowers (1875) reported the fatal illness and autopsy of a 30-year-old man with a previous history of rheumatic fever (Figure 1.7)[55] He was unconscious when admitted to the hospital, and it was later determined that he had suffered simultaneous embolism of the central retinal and middle cerebral arteries. "The heart was much diseased. The mitral orifice was thickened and roughened, and calcareous on its auricular surface. Old clots were contained on the auricular appendices and in the apex of the right ventricle." The left retinal artery and the left middle cerebral artery contained clots. This may be the earliest description of simultaneous cerebral and ophthalmic embolism due to disease.

During the nineteenth century it was generally accepted that cerebral hemorrhage was the consequence of rupture of diseased cerebral arteries.

Figure 1.7. SIR WILLIAM GOWERS
(From Haymaker W, Schiller F: *The Founders of Neurology*, 2nd Edition, 1970. Courtesy of Dr. Foster Kennedy, New York, and Charles C Thomas, Publisher, Springfield, IL)

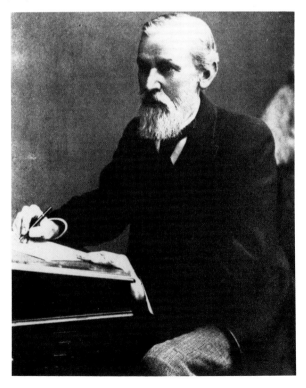

Charcot (1866) and Bouchard (1872), however, put forth the hypothesis that apoplectic hemorrhages were due to minute dilatations on the cerebral arteries.[56] They called these dilatations "miliary aneurysms" and their rupture was thought to be the cause of the hemorrhage. This process was not considered by them to be related to atherosclerosis.

In 1875, Broadbent reported a case of absence of pulses in both radial arteries in a 50-year-old patient with ascites and emphysema.[57] At autopsy, the orifices of the innominate and left carotid arteries (at their origin in the arch of the aorta) were close together. The lumen of the innominate was very small and the wall rigid with an atheromatous plaque. Immediately above the constriction, the innominate resumed its usual size and was elastic. The left vertebral artery "sprang from the arch of the aorta close to the origin of the subclavian, the orifice of which was narrowed to the size of a crowquill by the proximity of the vertebral." The orifice was rigid with atheroma, but the artery beyond that was full and healthy. The "constriction at the mouth of each of these two arteries with a larger elastic part beyond would neutralize the pulsatile movement of the blood." The narrowing "cut off the arteries from the general expansile movement of the aorta, as it would only permit the passage of a small stream of blood insufficient to distend them; this stream would be rendered more or less continuous by the pressure of the aorta" and "any inequality in the propulsion would be further diminished by the large elastic part of the vessel." The "occurrence of atheroma in an advanced stage at the narrowed orifices, while it was almost entirely absent elsewhere, illustrates the effects of strain" in producing atheromatous disease. There is always stress of the arterial wall where the aorta gives off its major branches and the blood stream is diverted. Atheromata develop here earlier than elsewhere and the stress is greatly increased by the constriction, "just as there is a more rapid current and greater wear and tear of the banks at a narrow part of a river."

Penzoldt (1881) reported a case of thrombosis of the right common carotid artery. The initial symptom was sudden blindness, and the sight in the right eye remained permanently defective with atrophy of the disc. Later, a left hemiplegia developed. Autopsy showed complete thrombosis of the right common carotid artery with a large area of softening in the right hemisphere.[58]

In a textbook published in 1885, Sir William Gowers presents a precise explanation of arterial occlusion:

Two pathological processes may cause the occlusion of an artery. A plug, from some distant source, may be carried into the vessel by the blood, and be arrested where the artery is narrower than the plug—"embolism"—or the clot may be formed in the artery by coagulation of the blood at the spot obstructed—"thrombosis." Embolism is the result of a morbid process elsewhere in the vascular system, commonly in the heart. Thrombosis is the result of a local disease of the artery, by which its calibre is narrowed and its inner surface is changed. The alteration in the wall of the vessel is usually the result of atheroma or of syphilitic disease. The process of occlusion is often aided by a change in the blood rendering it more prone to coagulate, or by a slower movement of the blood, giving it more time to coagulate.[59]

In 1896, Hill reported that ligation of both carotid and vertebral arteries in dogs and monkeys did not result in the death of the animals.[60] In 1898, Glück was far ahead of his time in replacing a segment of the common carotid artery with a vein graft in experimental animals.[38,61]

In Allbutt's *A System of Medicine* (1899), there is a description of embolism from the heart or from "diseased and roughened" arteries supplying the brain. The author noted that "in a number of cases recovery from the paralysis which follows embolism is both rapid and complete."[62,63] The concept of embolism to the eye or brain antedates even the first clear descriptions of transient ischemic attacks (TIAs). In fact, during the nineteenth century, there was considerable interest in both the clinical and pathological features of embolism, but these were for the most part disregarded during the first half of the twentieth century. Excellent descriptions of embolism from the heart can be found in the reports of several authors[55,64,65] and of embolism from the extracranial arteries in articles by others.[66,67,68]

The belief that occlusive disease of the extracranial blood vessels could be responsible for neurological symptoms was first proposed by Chiari (1905).[67] He emphasized the frequency of atherosclerosis in the region of the carotid bifurcation, believing that such lesions cause cerebral symptoms from atheromatous embolization. Chiari stressed the importance of examining at autopsy the cervical portions of carotid arteries in all patients dying from stroke. His interest was stimulated by a case of cerebral embolism in which no source of embolic material could be found. He finally opened the carotid vessels in their entire length and in one carotid sinus found thrombus material deposited on an atherosclerotic ulcer. The depression in the thrombus from which the embolic plug had separated could be identified. Chiari then examined 400 cases and in 7 cases observed gross parietal thrombosis in the region of the carotid bifurcation. In 4 of these cases cerebral embolism had occurred, the source of the embolism being the carotid sinus.

In another textbook published in 1906, Sir William Gowers stated:

Most cases of acute softening of the brain are due to the arrest of the blood supply by occlusion of an artery. . . . The sudden obstruction of a large vessel, however produced, frequently entails a distinct apoplectic attack. . . . In atheromatous thrombosis, focal symptoms, especially hemiplegia, come on before coma.[34]

Takayasu (1908), an ophthalmologist, described examination of a 21-year-old woman seen because of decreasing vision.[69] The retinal blood vessels contained "lumps" here and there, which were seen to move from day to day. In discussion, a colleague, Dr. Onishi, said that he had a similar patient but the "peculiar thing about this patient was that no radial pulses were felt no matter how hard we tried, and the arms were cold."[70] "Pulseless disease" was later named for Takayasu. In 1946 Frøvig wrote, "It would not be quite correct to speak of a syndrome of bilateral obliteration of the common carotid artery. A better term would be the syndrome arising from obliteration of the vessels branching off from the aortic arch."[71] This prompted use of the term "aortic arch syndrome."

In 1914, J. Ramsay Hunt, in an article considered to be another historical landmark in the recognition of the causes of cerebral ischemia, emphasized that strokes could be caused by extracranial occlusion of cerebral arteries (Figure 1.8). He described the syndrome of internal carotid occlusion and prefaced his paper with the following observations:

The object of the present study is to emphasize the importance of obstructive lesions of the main arteries of the neck in the causation of softening of the brain, and more especially to urge the routine examination of these vessels in all cases presenting cerebral symptoms of vascular origin. In other words, the writer would advocate the same attitude of mind toward this group of cases as towards intermittent claudication, gangrene, and other vascular symptoms of the extremities, and never omit a detailed examination of the main arterial stem.[72]

In the paper he stated that the neck arteries should be checked for "a possible diminution or absence of pulsation," and added, "I would also particularly emphasize the occurrence of unilateral vascular changes, pallor, or atrophy of the disk with contralateral hemiplegia in obstruction of the carotid artery."[72]

Unfortunately, the findings of Chiari and Hunt received little attention for about forty years. During this time, most areas of North America required that bodies be embalmed before burial. Undertakers insisted on having intact carotid arteries in the neck so that they would be available for injection. Therefore, autopsy examination rarely included dissection of the cervical carotid arteries. Once carotid arteriography had been de-

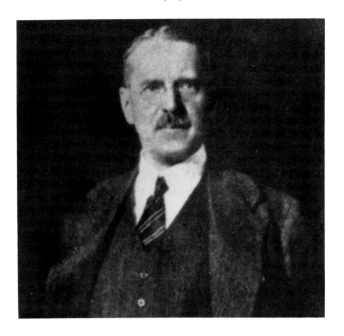

Figure 1.8. JAMES RAMSAY HUNT
(From Centennial Anniversary Volume of the American Neurological Association, 1875–1975. Courtesy of Springer Publishing Co., New York)

veloped and the condition of the common and internal carotid arteries could be ascertained in the living patient without resorting to surgical exploration, attention was again directed to obstructive lesions in the neck vessels.

References

1. Garrison FH: History of Neurology. Revised and enlarged by McHenry LC, Jr., Springfield, IL, Charles C Thomas, 1969.

2. Clarke E: Apoplexy in the Hippocratic writings. Bull Hist Med 37:301–314, 1963.

3. Ilberg G: Das neurologisch-psychiatrische wissen und können des Aretaeus von Kappa-dokien. Ztschr f d ges Neurol 86:227, 1923.

4. Drabkin IE: Caelius Aurelianus: On Acute Diseases and on Chronic Diseases. Chicago, University of Chicago Press, 1950.

5. Singer C: Vesalius on the Human Brain. London, Oxford University Press, 1952.

6. Vesalius A: De Humani Corpis Fabrica. Basileae, J. Oporini, 1543.

7. Willis T: Cerebri Anatome: Cui Accessit Nervorum Descriptio et Usus. Londini, J. Flesher, 1664.

8. Meyer A, Hierons R: Observations on the history of the circle of Willis. Med Hist 6:119–130, 1962.

9. Symonds C: The circle of Willis. Brit Med J 1:119–124, 1955.

10. Casserio G: Tabulae Anatomicae. Frankfurt, Daniel Buiretius, 1632.

11. Vesling J: Syntagma Anatomicum, Locis Plurimus Actum, Emendatum, Novisque Iconibus Diligenter Exornatum. Patavii, Pauli Frambotti Bibliopolae, 1647.

12. Wepfer JJ: Observationes Anatomicae, ex Cadaveribus Eorum, quos Sustulit Apoplexia, cum Exercitatione de Ejus Loco Affecto. Schaffhausen, Joh. Caspari Suteri, 1658.

13. Fields WS, Bruetman ME, Weibel J: Collateral Circulation of the Brain. Baltimore, Williams and Wilkins, 1965.

14. Nymman G: De Apoplexia Tractus, 2nd ed. Wittebergae, J.W. Fincelii, 1670.

15. Donley JE: John James Wepfer, a Renaissance student of apoplexy. Bull John Hopkins Hosp 20:1, 1909.

16. Fischer H: Johann Jakob Wepfer (1620–1695), ein Beitrage zur Medizingeschichte des 17 Jahrhunderts. Zurich, Rudolf, 1931.

17. Thomas HM: Decussation of the pyramids: An historical inquiry. Bull Johns Hopkins Hosp 21:304, 1910.

18. Mistichelli D: Trattato dell Apoplessia. Roma, A. de Rossi alla Piazza di Ceri, 1709.

19. Bayle F: Tractatus de Apoplexia. Toulouse, B. Guillemette, 1677.

20. Jandolo M: La struttura e la funzione nervosa in una lezione inedita di G. B. Morgagni. Pag Stor Med 3:10, 1959.

21. Morgagni GB: De Sedibus, et Causis Morborum per Anatomen Indagatis Libri Quinque. Vienna, ex typographica Remondiana, 1761.

22. Di Giacomo V: A case of Takayasu's disease occurred over two hundred years ago. Angiology 35:750–754, 1984.

23. Baillie M: The Morbid Anatomy of Some of the Most Important Parts of the Human Body. London, J. Johnson and G. Nicol, 1793.

24. Heberden W: Epilepsy, head-ache, palsy and apoplexy, and St. Vitus dance. In Commentaries on the History and Cure of Diseases. London, T. Payne, 1802.

25. Hunter J: (Cited by J. Kobler) The Reluctant Surgeon. Garden City, NY, Doubleday, 1960.

26. Home E: An account of Mr. Hunter's method of performing the operation for popliteal aneurism. Lond Med J 7:391, 1786.

27. Romano J, Merritt HH: The singular affection of Gaspard Vieusseux: An early description of the lateral medullary syndrome. Bull Hist Med 9:72–79, 1941.

28. Linnaeus C von: Glömska af alla substantive och i synnerhet namm. K Svenska Wetensk Akad Handl 6:116, 1745.

29. Viets HR: Aphasia as described by Linnaeus and as painted by Ribera. Bull Hist Med 13:328–333, 1943.

30. Swieten G von: Of the Apoplexy, Palsy and Epilepsy. Commentaries upon the Aphorisms of Dr. Herman Boerhaave. London, John and Paul Knapton, 1754.

31. Cheyne J: Cases of Apoplexy and Lethargy with Observations on Comatose Patients. London, Thomas Underwood, 1812.

32. Cooke J: A Treatise on Nervous Diseases. Vol. 1. On Apoplexy. London, Longman, Hurst, Rees, Orme & Brown, 1820.

33. Rostan L: Recherches sur le ramollissement du cerveau; ouvrage dans lequel on s'efforce de distinguer les diverses affections de ce viscère par des signes caractéristiques. Paris, Béchet jeune, 1823.

34. Gowers WR: A Manual of Diseases of the Nervous System, 2nd ed., Vol. II. Philadelphia, Blakiston's Sons and Co., pp. 421–449, 1906.

35. Abercrombie J: Pathological and Practical Researches on Diseases of the Brain and Spinal Cord. Edinburgh, Waugh and Innes, 1828.

36. Carswell R: Pathological Anatomy: Illustrations of the Elementary Forms of Disease. London, Longman and Co., 1838.

37. Virchow R: Archiv für Pathologische Anatomie und Physiologie und für Klinische Medizin. Vol. 1. Berlin, Druck und Verlag von G. Reimer, 1847.

38. Robicsek F: The medical history of extracranial cerebrovascular disease. In Extracranial Cerebrovascular Disease: Diagnosis and Management, Robicsek F (ed), New York, Macmillan, pp. 5–18, 1986.

39. Keevil JJ: David Fleming and the operation for ligation of the carotid artery. Brit J Surg 37:92–95, 1949.

40. Cooper A: Some experiments and observations on tying the carotid and vertebral arteries, and the pneumogastric, phrenic, and sympathetic nerves. Guy's Hosp Rep 1:457, 1836.

41. Chevers N: Remarks on the effects of obliteration of the carotid arteries upon the cerebral circulation. London Med Gaz 1:1140, 1845.

42. Davy J: Researches, Physiological and Anatomic, Vol. 1, London, Smith Elder & Co., p. 426, 1839.

43. Ellis J: Case of gunshot wound attended with secondary hemorrhage in which both carotid arteries were tied at an interval of four and a half days. NY J Med and Surg 5:187–189, 1845.

44. Rich NM, Spencer FC: Historical aspects of vascular trauma. In Vascular Trauma. Philadelphia, W.B. Saunders, p. 6, 1978.

45. Burrows G: On Disorders of the Cerebral Circulation and on the Connection Between Affections of the Brain and Disease of the Heart, London, Longman, Brown, Green and Longmans, 1846.

46. Durand-Fardel M: Traité du ramollissement du cerveau. Paris, J.B. Baillière, 1843.

47. Román GC: Les lacunes cérébrales: Étude clinique et neuropathologique de 100 cas. Mémoire pour le titre d'Assistant Étranger. Paris, Faculté de Médecine Pitié-Salpêtrière, 1975.

48. Dechambre A: Mémoire sur la curabilité du ramollissement cérébral. Gaz Méd Paris 6:305–314, 1838.

49. Román GC: The original description of lacunes. Neurology 36:85, 1986.

50. Gull WW: Case of occlusion of the innominate and left carotid. Guy's Hosp Rep 1:12, 1855.

51. Savory WS: Case of a young woman in whom the main arteries of both upper extremities and of the left side of the neck were throughout completely obliterated. Med Chir Trans London 39:205–219, 1856.

52. Gurdjian ES and Gurdjian ES: History of occlusive cerebrovascular disease. I. From Wepfer to Moniz. Arch Neurol 36:340–343, 1979.

53. Virchow R: Thrombose und Embolie: Gefässenzündung und Septische Infektion. In Gesammelte Abhandlungen zur wissen schaftlichen Medicin. Frankfurt a. M., Meidinger, Sohn und Co., pp. 219–732, 1856.

54. Kussmaul A: Zwei Fälle von spontaner allmäliger Verschliessung grosser Halsarterienstamme. Deutsch Klin 24:461–465, 1872.

55. Gowers WR: On a case of simultaneous embolism of central retinal and middle cerebral arteries. Lancet 2:794–796, 1875.

56. Bouchard C: A Study of Some Points in the Pathology of Cerebral Hemorrhage. London, Simpkin, Marshall and Co., 1872.

57. Broadbent WH: Absence of pulsation in both radial arteries, vessels being full of blood. Trans Clin Soc London, 8:165, 1875.

58. Penzoldt F: Über Thrombose (autochthone oder embolische) der Carotis. Deutsches Arch f klin Med 28:80, 1881.

59. Gowers WR: Diagnosis of Diseases of the Brain and Spinal Cord. New York, William Wood, pp. 164–165, 1885.

60. Hill L: The Physiology and Pathology of the Cerebral Circulation: an Experimental Research. London, J and A Churchill, 1896.

61. Glück T: Die moderne Chirurgie des circulations Apparates. Berl Klin 129:1–29, 1898.

62. Taylor J: Occlusion of cerebral vessels. In A System of Medicine, Vol. VII, T. C. Allbutt (ed.), London, Macmillan, pp. 560–576, 1899.

63. Welch WH: Embolism. In A System of Medicine, Vol. VI, T. C. Allbutt (ed.), London, Macmillan, pp. 228–285, 1899.

64. von Graefe A: Über embolie der arteria centralis retinae als ursacht plotzlicher erblindung. Graefes Arch Ophthalmol 5:136–157, 1859.

65. Coats G: Obstruction of the central artery of the retina. Royal London Ophthal Hosp Rep 16:262–305, 1905.

66. Knapp H: Über Verstopfung der blutgefässe des auges. Graefes Arch Ophthalmol 14:207–251, 1868.

67. Chiari H: Über das Verhalten des Tielungswinkels der Carotis communis bei der Endarteritis chronica deformans. Verhandl d deutsch path Gesellsch 9:326–330, 1905.

68. Fisher CM: Occlusion of the internal carotid artery. Arch Neurol Psychiat 65:346–377, 1951.

69. Takayasu M: A case with peculiar changes of the central retinal vessels. Acta Soc Ophth Jap 12:554, 1908.

70. Translated in Judge RD, Currier RD, Gracie WA, et al: Takayasu's arteritis and the aortic arch syndrome. Am J Med 32:379–392, 1962.

71. Frøvig AG: Bilateral obliteration of the common carotid artery: Thromboangiitis obliterans? Acta Psychiat Neurol suppl 39:3–79, 1946.

72. Hunt JR: The role of the carotid arteries in the causation of vascular lesions of the brain, with remarks on certain special features of the symptomatology. Am J M Sc 147:704–713, 1914.

2

Collateral Circulation

Erasistratus is given credit for introducing the term "anastomosis" in the third century B.C., to describe hypothetical connections between veins and arteries.[1] Gradually it has come to designate not only arteriovenous, but interarterial and intervenous connections.[2]

Quiring states:

> Anastomoses are the basis for collateral circulation or, stated differently, collateral vessels represent anastomoses of sufficient caliber to supply the vascular requirements in event of injury to the primary vessels. Such secondary channels are developments from the original embryonic capillary network. This network, then, is a reserve or an insurance against total loss of a structure when its usual blood supply is restricted or obliterated.[2]

Richard Lower, the physiologist and colleague of Thomas Willis, wrote a letter to Robert Boyle in June 1668:

> . . . the carotidal and vertebral arteries have so many anastomoses, so divinely contrived inside the dura matter, before they go up into the brain . . . that if three arteries were quite obstructed, the fourth would convey blood into all parts of the brain and cerebellum, sufficient enough for life and motion.[3]

Frederik Ruysch (1638–1731), a Dutch anatomist, has been called "the apostle of the injection method." He injected various organs and noted specific types of networks and ramifications in many parts of the body (Figure 2.1). His success in injection technique led him to the erroneous conclusion that, "The tissues are nothing but vascular networks variously arranged."[2] Ruysch was the first to demonstrate the subarachnoid arterial anastomoses between the major cerebral vessels (1724).[4] Heubner[5] (1874) described anastomoses between cortical arteries over the surface of the

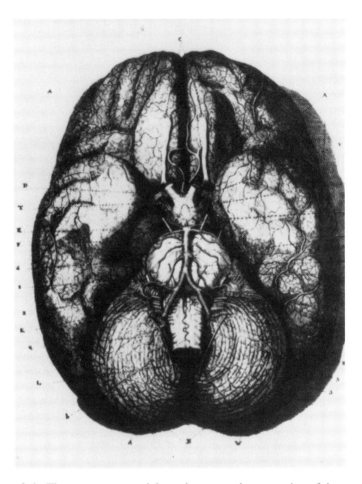

Figure 2.1. The most accurate eighteenth-century demonstration of the cerebral vasculature is this injection specimen prepared by Frederik Ruysch (1724). The arteries at the base of the brain and their branchings are shown for the first time. (From Garrison FH: *History of Neurology.* Revised and enlarged by McHenry LC, Jr., 1969. Courtesy of Charles C Thomas, Publisher, Springfield, IL)

brain. He found that if one of the cerebral arteries was ligated close to its origin from the circle of Willis and a colored fluid injected into the distal branches, all of the cerebral arteries could be filled through a complete network of pial vessels.[6] It has been suggested by Van der Eecken and Adams (1953) "that the presence of encephalic meningeal anastomoses may be a vestigial remnant of the primordial plexus from which all the brain vessels are derived."[7] They further postulated that "such an arrangement of meningeal anastomoses, by providing variability of distribution of blood, assures a greater constancy of supply under conditions of health and disease."[7]

Antyllus may have been the first to note that ligation of an artery did not necessarily result in loss of the part served by that vessel. Some 15 centuries later (as described in Chapter 1), the great surgeon John Hunter was surprised to find that ligation of the main artery of a stag's antler did not interrupt its growth. Furthermore, he discovered that in time there was prodigious growth of vessels which bypassed the ligated artery. He stated in 1785, "All the uses arising from the anastomosing of the vessels are, perhaps, not yet perfectly understood, general reasons can, I think, be assigned for them, but these will not apply in all cases, it is something, therefore, more than we are yet acquainted with."[8] With the rise of surgery and its interference with the circulatory channels, the problem of anastomoses and collateral circulation became a practical one.

Carotid Artery Ligation

According to Robicsek (see Chapter 1) the first report of operative ligation of the common carotid artery was that of Ambrose Paré in 1552. His patient, however, developed aphasia and hemiplegia. Elective ligation of the common carotid artery with survival was performed by Hebenstreit and reported in 1793.

The earliest recorded carotid artery ligation with a detailed account of the procedure appears to have been performed by David Fleming, a naval surgeon, on October 9, 1803.[9] On that day a servant on the ship attempted suicide by cutting his own throat. He was bleeding freely and, unable to move him, Fleming ligated the bleeding vessels on the spot; the man was pulseless. The wound, 4 inches long, had divided "the trachea between the thyroid and cricoid cartilages, the two superior thyroid arteries, the internal jugular vein, and grazed the outer and muscular coats of the carotid artery." Fleming then brought the divided parts into contact, securing the patient's head well forward on the chest. Convalescence was satisfactory until October 17 when, during a paroxysm of coughing, the carotid artery burst and "torrents of blood issued from the mouth and nose."[9] Fleming's attempts to secure the artery through the wound failed owing to the friable state of the vessel, and he therefore cut down on it below the wound. He "had never heard of such an operation being performed," but the patient was now *in extremis*.[9] After tying the common carotid artery, the patient made an uneventful recovery. By October 22 he was able to swallow. On October 24, Fleming removed the ligature by dissecting through healthy granulation tissue.

John Abernathy (1804) reported a carotid ligation, but gave no exact date for the operation which he performed at St. Bartholomew's Hospital. He ligated the left common carotid artery of a man who had been gored in the neck by a cow. The patient died 30 hours later with various cerebral symptoms, which can today be attributed to other causes, but which Abernathy interpreted as the result of the operation.[9] He wrote:

> Though the stopping of the blood supply to the brain did not for several hours produce any apparent derangement in the functions of the organ, yet such a state was gradually occasioned by it, and which was attended like the effects of concussion of the brain, with inflammation.[9,10]

Astley Cooper is generally cited as the first surgeon to ligate the carotid artery. His first patient (1805) had a large aneurysm of the right carotid artery. She died of suppuration and fatal compression of the larynx and trachea 20 days after ligation of the vessel. In 1808, Cooper ligated the common carotid because of an aneurysm about the size of an egg at the bifurcation. The man lived 13 years, dying of cerebral hemorrhage on the same side.[11]

Circle of Willis

In 1664, Willis published his *Cerebri Anatome,* in which he described the arterial anastomosis at the base of the brain that has since borne his name (Figure 2.2).[12] He performed injection experiments on cadavers and in 1684 wrote:

> Let the Carotidick Arteries be laid bare on either side of the Cervix on the hinder part of the head, so that their little tubes or Pipes, about half an inch long, may be exhibited together to the sight; then let a dyed liquor, and contained in a large Squirt or Pipe, be injected upwards in the trunk of one side, after once or twice injecting, you shall see the tincture or dyed liquor to descend from the other side by the trunk of the opposite Artery.[13]

As a result of the conclusions drawn from this experiment, for 250 years physicians believed that it was the function of the circle of Willis to equalize the blood supply to all parts of the brain.[14] However, Kramer (1912) studied conditions in living dogs and monkeys and stated that the carotid and vertebral blood flows do not mix, unless there is a reduced

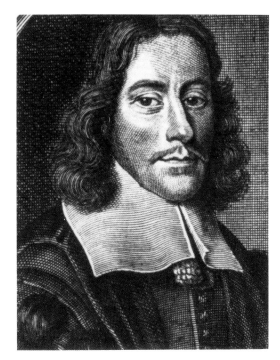

Figure 2.2. THOMAS WILLIS
(From Garrison FH: *History of Neurology.* Revised and enlarged by McHenry LC, Jr., 1969. Courtesy of Charles C Thomas, Publisher, Springfield, IL)

pressure due to an obstruction on the side of the circle opposite the injection.[14] Kramer appears to have been the first to report physiologic experiments. He showed that both the carotid and vertebral arteries have distinct territories of supply and concluded that the circle was an antero-posterior anastomosis, which "under physiological conditions does not permit the mingling of the bloodstreams." He noted that after carotid injection, the dye stopped at the posterior communicating artery, where there was a deadpoint, "the place where the opposing streams from the carotid and vertebral arteries meet, and, the pressure being equal, the streams do not mix." McDonald and Potter (1951) showed that each vertebral artery supplies just the ipsilateral half of the brainstem, and that the deadpoint between carotid and vertebral circulations can move rapidly due to pressure changes in these systems.[15]

After the introduction of cerebral arteriography, interest in the cerebral circulation in living man was stimulated and the findings confirmed Kramer's statements. If one carotid is injected, the carotid system of that side only is outlined; very little of the medium leaks into the opposite side or into the posterior cerebral arteries. Blood leaving the carotid and basilar arteries passes directly into the main branches of these vessels, the communicating arteries merely constituting an anastomosis in their course with little influence on the main stream.[16] Rogers (1947) stated:

> Thus, the circle of Willis should not be looked upon as a distributor or equalizing station or booster mechanism for the cerebral blood supply, but merely as an anastomosis. The great value of an anastomosis is its potential effect as a shunt capable of opening up and playing an important part should one of the main vessels be occluded.[16]

Rogers appears to be one of the earliest investigators to outline the collateral function of the circle.

Although the circle of Willis is present to some degree in all human brains, it shows considerable variation. In fact, it is estimated that the "normal" circle exists in less than 50% of cases. Anatomical dissimilarities, therefore, are not truly abnormal and need not be associated with any inadequacy of circulation.[17] The circle does, however, represent the best potential source of collateral flow between the two internal carotid arteries or between the basilar artery and either the right or left carotid. Whether the circle can provide adequate collateral flow depends on the caliber of its vessels.[17]

In some patients the collateral pathways, especially those of the circle of Willis, are not developed well enough to protect the brain from ischemia.[18] In a Japanese study of 400 autopsies, Kameyama and Okinaka (1963) reported that an embryonic derivation of the posterior cerebral artery from the internal carotid was observed two to three times more frequently in Japanese than in Americans or Europeans and that it was found more frequently in brains with infarction.[19] This latter observation had also been made by Alpers and Berry (1963).[20] They found that, in cases of cerebral softening (cerebral infarction), the posterior communicating arteries were string-like in 38%, compared to 22% in the controls. The clinical importance of anomalies of the circle was stressed by Saphir (1935), who stated that a good collateral anastomosis between the carotid and vertebral arteries through the posterior communicating artery would be essential in diffuse atherosclerosis.[18,21] He said, "An interference with the passage of blood through the circle of Willis does not make itself manifest until the circulation through the internal carotid and vertebral arteries is impaired."[21] Meyer et al. (1954) found that the extent of cerebral ischemia resulting from occlusion of one or both carotid arteries in the monkey was directly related to the size of the posterior communicating arteries.[22]

It had long been recognized that abnormalities of the circle of Willis might be related in some way to cerebral softenings.[20] Leidy (1891) reported a case with multiple cerebral softenings in which the anterior communicating artery was "less than a line" (2.12 mm) in length and in which the posterior communicating artery on the left side was increased in diameter (3 lines or 6.36 mm), while that of the right side was no thicker than a hair.[20,23] He suggested the possibility that the cerebral softenings were connected with the anomalous circle of Willis but failed to offer a clear idea of their relationship.

Extracranial Occlusive Disease

The most common cause of stenosis in the major arteries is atherosclerosis, usually involving a bifurcation area. Before total obstruction takes place, the lumen of the vessel gradually becomes narrowed by deposition of subintimal atheromatous material. When the lumen is compromised to the point where blood flow is so retarded that thrombosis occurs, the viability of the tissue normally supplied by the primary vessel becomes dependent on the collateral circulation.[6] It has often been stated that if this process of narrowing is gradual rather than abrupt, there is more likelihood that adequate collateral flow will be established. However, in recent years, that belief has been disputed. Eikelboom (1981) wrote:

> Whether gradual mechanical occlusion gives less chance of ischemic complications than sudden occlusion, because the collateral circulation would be able to develop, remains a question. The cooperative study (Nishioka,[24] 1966) gives no statistic proof about the advantage of gradual occlusion. It must be taken into consideration that hemodynamic changes only take place with an occlusion of about 80–90% of the area of the vessel lumen. Brice et al.[25] (1964) even conclude that it is not possible to obtain a gradual and progressive reduction in pressure and flow.[18]

Brice et al. found that the human carotid artery must be very severely narrowed before there is any change of pressure gradient or of flow. They stated:

> It is very improbable that a stenosis is significant if its minimal cross-section is greater than 5 sq. mm, even if it occupies the whole length of the internal carotid, and this is also true for several stenoses in series; it

is very probable that a stenosis is significant if its minimal cross-section is less than 2 sq. mm, however short it is.[25]

Thus, they believed that many stenoses classified as "severe" almost certainly had negligible effects on resistance. In the past, many authors have classified stenoses greater than 50% as "severe."

According to Fields et al. (1965) when thrombosis occurs in the cervical portion of the internal carotid artery, collateral circulation is established through one of the following routes: (1) from the cross-filling through the anterior segment of the circle of Willis via the anterior cerebral and anterior communicating arteries; (2) from the basilar artery circulation via the ipsilateral posterior communicating artery; (3) from the external carotid artery branches via the ophthalmic artery; and (4) from the external carotid branches via the carotico-tympanic arteries.[6] When the common carotid artery becomes occluded, the major collateral inflow comes from three sources: (1) from the branches of the contralateral external carotid artery; (2) from the branches on the side of the obstruction provided by the thyrocervical and costocervical trunks of the subclavian artery; and (3) from the ipsilateral vertebral artery via the external carotid arteries.[6]

Kelly and Strandness (1969) wrote:

> Although from a purely anatomic point of view it is possible to outline all the potential collateral pathways, this has very little meaning relative to the function of these vessels in response to acute or chronic occlusions. The greatest test of a collateral pathway is its response to an acute obstruction of a major artery. If the vessels are capable of maintaining viability of the area supplied following an acute occlusion, it is almost certain that with time collateral flow will improve even further.[26]

The circle of Willis is generally considered to be the most important source of collateral flow in extracranial cerebrovascular disease.

Treating intracranial aneurysms by ligating either the common or internal carotid artery has provided important data on the immediate response of collateral arteries. Love and Dart (1967) reported that 6 of 15 patients with ligation of the internal carotid artery suffered hemiparesis, as compared to 1 of 17 patients undergoing interruption of the common carotid.[27] The number of potential collateral pathways is greater as the location of the obstruction is more proximal.[18] Ischemic complication rates for occlusion of the internal versus the common carotid artery, reported in the Cooperative Study of Intracranial Aneurysms and Subarachnoid Hemorrhage, were 49% and 28%, respectively.[24]

The adequacy of collateral pathways is not only dependent on the anatomy of the network but also on the condition of the vessels. With aging, the arterial wall undergoes degenerative changes.[18] The number of atherosclerotic obstructions is also important. The more lesions, the less adequate the collateral circulation will be.[28] Toole (1966) said, "The production of symptoms in patients with occlusive forms of cerebral vascular disease depends to a large extent upon the matrix of vessels laid down within the first 90 days of intra-uterine life and upon the atheromatous material deposited in these vessels during the next ensuing years."[28]

Vessels of older persons may lose their capacity to dilate because of atrophy of elastic tissue and other degenerative changes.[18] Kunihiko et al. (1975) have shown that the increase in collateral circulation following a carotid occlusion was poorer in patients with cerebrovascular disease and/or hypertension than in healthy younger persons.[29] Also, autopsy studies have taught us that, as a rule, the circle of Willis is not better developed in cases of cerebrovascular disease, but probably poorer.[18] Meyer et al. (1965) stated, "The capacity of the cerebral collateral circulation appears to decrease with advancing age and cerebrovascular disease."[30] Eikelboom wrote, "Whether adaptation of the circle of Willis can take place or not is an individual variable. In some people it is adequate and in others it seems to be not possible at all."[18]

Bilateral Carotid Artery Occlusion

Before the 1950s complete bilateral internal carotid occlusion had been considered to be incompatible with normal brain function. Frøvig (1946) related the case history of a 21-year-old girl with complete obstruction of both carotids, possibly due to thromboangiitis obliterans.[31] A vertebral artery was hypertrophied and supplied blood to the anterior cerebral vessels, as was demonstrated by angiography. Resected segments of the carotids revealed complete obstruction. She had multiple symptoms, including visual problems, drop attacks, and frequent ischemic episodes. However, she was alive (in a nursing home) at the time of the report.

Fisher (1954) reported that of 432 consecutive autopsies, bilateral occlusion occurred in 11 cases.[32] Eisenbrey et al. (1955) encountered three cases; one died but the other two were functioning with some neurologic deficits.[33] Batley (1955) cited two cases of bilateral carotid thrombosis.[34] A 50-year-old male whose vertebral angiogram showed filling of the right middle cerebral artery as well as the normal posterior cerebral arteries was followed for nine months and was doing fine at his work as a bricklayer. A 56-year-old male was first seen with right hemiplegia and dysphasia. Angiography showed cerebral vessels that filled from the vertebrals. A year later he was able to walk a little, but he died a week after that examination (cause unknown).

Clarke and Harrison (1956) detailed the progressive dementia of a patient who, at autopsy, had bilateral obstruction of the internal carotid arteries in the cavernous sinuses due to giant-cell arteritis.[35] The authors reviewed all cases of bilateral occlusion in the literature (69 patients) and found that only 10% had severe mental changes. Gurdjian et al. (1960) reported 9 bilateral occlusions among 131 patients with complete carotid occlusion.[36] These cases were proved either by angiography or surgical exploration, but detailed histories of the 9 cases were not included. Groch and colleagues (1960) described the case history of a patient who was living 3 years after the diagnosis of bilateral complete carotid occlusion.[37] He had not had a recurrent stroke or mental deterioration. A second person with the same diagnosis died 7 weeks after the onset of symptoms.

The largest published series in these early years was by Fields et al. (1961), who presented specific details on 16 patients with complete bilateral occlusion of the carotid system.[38] Of these, 15 were males, 1 female; they were between the ages of 45 and 68 years. In reviewing their symptoms and signs, several patterns became evident: (1) 6 had adequate collateral circulation and minimal deficit; (2) 7 had impaired or absent collateral circulation and severe deficit; and (3) 3 had prompt surgery to restore circulation after an acute occlusion with severe deficit and uncertain collateral. There were 6 deaths in this series, but only 3 could be attributed to central nervous system lesions resulting from impaired circulation. In 2 patients, death resulted from cardiac disease, and in 1, from a cerebellar neoplasm. Of the 10 surviving patients, 6 were functioning remarkably well and returned to their usual occupations. Of the remaining 4 patients, 1 was demented, and 3 suffered from varying degrees of motor and/or language impairment.

In 1963, Doniger reported a case of bilateral complete carotid and basilar artery occlusion with the patient having only a minimal deficit.[39] This 48-year-old black woman experienced visual phenomena (suggestive of episodic bilateral occipital lobe dysfunction) and two attacks of right hemiparesis. She recovered spontaneously with residual deficit consisting only of mild visual field defect. Reuter and Newton (1964) described a relatively asymptomatic 49-year-old man with angiographically proved atherosclerotic occlusion of both common and internal carotids and the right vertebral artery.[40] Cerebral circulation depended on a small left vertebral artery and well developed collateral channels from thyrocervical and costocervical trunks supplying the external carotids and the right vertebral artery above the occlusion.

Bilateral complete carotid occlusion places an arduous strain on collateral vessels in the body's effort to maintain cerebral function. When this auxiliary or reserve circulation proves to be sufficient, individuals may continue in good health at their regular occupations. As stressed by Fields et al.:

> All patients in whom total occlusion of long duration is found in one carotid system should have arteriographic study of the contralateral carotid. Removal of a stenotic lesion of the latter may prevent a subsequent catastrophe.[38]

Basilar Artery Occlusion

Cravioto et al. (1958)[41] state that occluson of the basilar artery was first described by Kingston in 1842.[42] Other reports that appeared during the 1800s were mainly based on cases of syphilitic origin. In 1868, Hayem described pathologic changes in a case of occluded basilar artery but gave no clinical features.[43] Leyden (1882) reported two cases at autopsy, both revealing thrombotic occlusion of the basilar artery, probably due to syphilitic arteritis.[44] Leyden stressed that, of the arteries, the basilar is a favored site of syphilitic changes.[45]

Publications since 1930 have considered atherosclerosis to be the main etiologic factor. This was emphasized by Lhermitte and Trelles (1934)[46] and by Kubik and Adams[47] in their landmark article appearing in 1946. Until the latter publication the diagnosis was made at autopsy in all cases. Kubik and Adams reported 18 cases with autopsy findings and 4 additional cases that recovered. They were the first to suggest the possibility of making the diagnosis during life. Their four recovered cases had symptoms sufficiently resembling those of the autopsied cases to make the diagnosis of basilar artery occlusion almost certain. Kubik and Adams provided clarification of the signs and symptoms of obstruction of the basilar artery and gave the most comprehensive account of the condition.

In 1947, Pratt-Thomas and Berger presented two postmortem cases of thrombosis of the basilar artery following chiropractic manipulation.[48] Biemond (1951) described four terminal cases of basilar artery occlusion.[49] Three deaths were attributed to thrombosis of the artery and one to brainstem infarction secondary to inadvertent clipping of the basilar artery during surgery. In 1953, Freeman et al. reported the acute onset of complete tetraplegia, facial diplegia, and pseudobulbar palsy in a 40-year-old man.[50] He achieved a marked degree of recovery. The authors diagnosed basilar artery occlusion on clinical findings, but the patient did not have angiography.

To our knowledge, arteriographic demonstration of basilar artery occlusion during life was first reported by Haugsted (1956).[45] He described two cases in which the diagnosis was made first on the basis of the clinical manifestations and later corroborated by percutaneous vertebral angiography. In the first case there was dense filling of the vertebral artery with contrast medium, while only traces of contrast were seen in the basilar artery; the posterior cerebral and superior cerebellar arteries were distinctly filled. This indicated incomplete occlusion of the basilar artery. In the second case angiograms were made after injection into the right common carotid artery. There were marked atheromatous changes in the carotid system. The posterior communicating arteries were filled, as were the two posterior cerebral arteries and the two superior cerebellar arteries, and a reflux was demonstrable into the basilar artery for about an inch. The patient died 48 hours after the angiogram, and autopsy showed marked sclerosis and complete thrombosis of the basilar artery.

Cravioto et al. (1958) described the clinical and pathologic findings in 14 cases, all confirmed at autopsy.[41] These cases were mainly males, past middle age, admitted to Bellevue Hospital between 1938–1956. Arteriosclerosis, frequently with hemorrhage and ulceration of atheromatous plaques, and, less commonly, embolism were the etiologic factors in these occlusions. Eight of their patients were in coma at the time of admission, six were alert and conscious but later progressively deteriorated, and all 14 died within 3 to 30 days following admission.

In 1962, Mount and Taveras reported ligation of the basilar artery in treatment of an aneurysm at the basilar bifurcation in a 25-year-old man:

> Since what appeared to be adequate collateral circulation was demonstrated arteriographically, the basilar artery was ligated between the origins of the posterior cerebral and the superior cerebellar arteries.[51]

One year after the operation, the only abnormal sign was nystagmus on lateral gaze to the left side. The man was asymptomatic and returned to his previous job of salesman.

Fields and colleagues (1966) described eight patients in whom segmental occlusion of the basilar artery was demonstrated arteriographically.[52] In all of these cases the vertebral artery circulation was defective because of congenital anomalies, atherosclerosis, or both, causing them to be more dependent on collateral circulation from the carotid system. Three of the four patients in whom the circle of Willis was asymmetrical had mild but permanent neurologic deficit. Two patients had normally functioning posterior communicating arteries bilaterally. One of them had no neurologic deficit and the other a minimal right hemiparesis of several years duration due to an old infarct in the left cerebral hemisphere. One patient with occlusive disease involving the cervical portion of the carotid artery became asymptomatic after carotid endarterectomy. Another patient with extensive occlusive disease involving both internal carotids and vertebral arteries was in a state of akinetic mutism. Her condition remained unchanged and was not improved by vertebral endarterectomy.

Since these early reports, there have been many subsequent articles on basilar artery occlusion. It has become apparent that the extent of neurologic deficit is dependent on the adequacy of collateral circulation; when collateral pathways are available and patent, maintenance of function is possible.

Evaluation of Potential Collateral Circulation

Among the various procedures that yield information regarding the efficiency of collateral circulation to the brain, carotid compression has the oldest history. Galen was aware of the relationship between the carotid artery and syncopal episodes, stating that the vessel was so named because when pressure was externally applied, it produced *karos,* or deep sleep.[53] At his time it was believed that this outcome was due to "compression of the sensitive nerves which lie near the arteries."[54,55] The ancient Assyrians reportedly used carotid pressure as a means of analgesia in their rites of circumcision.[56] The Persian Avicenna (980–1037) stated that when the carotid artery was ligated, sense and motion were lost.[55,57] If the carotid artery were temporarily obstructed, Valverdus noted that we immediately "grow stupid and fall asleep."[55,57]

By the late 1700s carotid compression was used as therapy for many complaints, such as mania, headache, vertigo, convulsions, hysteria, and palpitations of the heart.[55] Caleb Parry (1792) (Figure 2.3) noted that it caused a slowing of the heart and "almost immediately a sound sleep."[55,58] Later in the next century (1859) Kussmaul and Tenner reported that besides unconsciousness, convulsive movements may accompany ischemia of the brain from carotid compression when applied bilaterally.[55,59] Nauyn, who succeeded Kussmaul at Strassburg, found individual differences in reaction to the test and also found a relation with atherosclerosis and explained the effects by impairment of blood flow to the brain through the vertebral arteries and the circle of Willis.[54,55]

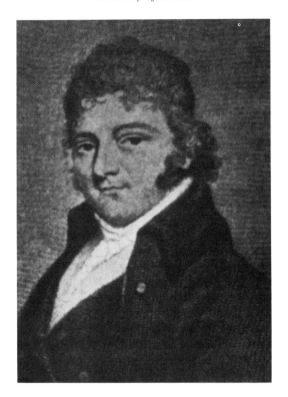

Figure 2.3. CALEB HILLIER PARRY
(An engraving by Philip Audinet from a miniature sketch by John Hay Bell,
1804. From Annals of Medical History 9:8, 1937. Courtesy of Lippincott, Harper
& Row, Publisher, Philadelphia. PA)

When he gave the President's address at the meeting of the American
Surgical Association in June 1910, Matas declared:

> The surgery of the vascular system bristles with problems which still await
> solution, but none appears to me more important or fundamental than the
> study of the collateral circulation in its behavior to occluded arteries and
> in the means of testing its efficiency or inefficiency before permanently
> obstructing the more important arterial channels of the circulation.[60]

Matas used carotid compression to determine the tolerance for ligation in
patients with intracranial carotid aneurysms and to enhance collaterals by
carrying out the test at frequent intervals (Figure 2.4). Matas had done
over 78 ligations and extirpations of common and internal carotid arteries

over a 25-year period and this experience had convinced him that the risk of fatal intracranial complication resulting from an insufficient collateral circulation should not be underestimated. He used aluminum bands, developed by Halsted, to occlude the vessels without injuring the vessel walls. These were applied under local anesthesia and could be removed quickly if untoward symptoms developed. The band could be left in place for 3 to 4 days before obliterative changes occurred in the intima; it could be used instead of ligature and left in permanently.[60]

During the present century, Hering (1927)[61] and Heymans (1929)[62] focused attention on a neural reflex mechanism in the carotid sinus to regulate blood flow to the brain.[55] Then, Weiss and Baker in 1933 clearly outlined the clinical syndrome associated with hyperactivity of the carotid sinus.[63] They described faintness, syncope, and convulsive movements

Figure 2.4. RUDOLPH MATAS
(From Postgraduate Medicine 34:A-129, December 1963, Courtesy of Postgraduate Medicine, Minneapolis, MN and Louisiana State Medical Society, New Orleans, LA)

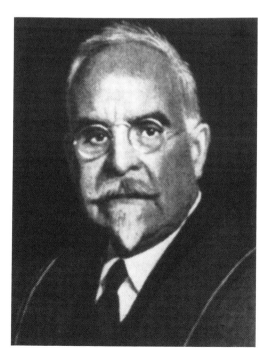

occurring as a result of carotid massage but detected no irreversible neurologic changes in the patients tested.[56] After it was recognized that, occasionally, patients have spontaneous episodes of syncope because of hypersensitivity of the carotid sinus, some physicians massaged the carotid sinus of every patient they examined. Not until 1941 was it recorded that irreversible neurologic damage could result from the maneuver.[56]

In that year, Marmor and Sapirstein reported the case of a 53-year-old patient whose pulse slowed immediately following carotid compression and he developed generalized clonic twitching and syncope.[64] Several minutes later he became unresponsive and manifested weakness of the limbs of the right side. Six hours later he had spasticity of all limbs. At necropsy, there were recent hemorrhagic infarcts of both frontal lobes. The vessels of the circle of Willis were moderately stenotic.[56]

Calverley and Millikan (1961) cited four cases from the Mayo Clinic with severe neurologic defects coincident with manipulation of carotid arteries.[56] They believed that even gentle pressure over the carotid is not without danger. They concluded that cerebral infarction may be produced by manual occlusion of the artery, by embolization of dislodged atheromatous material, and by local trauma to the vessel with subsequent thrombosis or formation of a dissecting aneurysm. It appeared probable that decrease in systemic blood pressure, bradycardia, and cerebral vasospasm were not the direct cause of complications.

Askey (1946) described seven patients having reactions from carotid sinus stimulation, including hemiplegia, dizziness, facial pallor, syncope, convulsions, numbness, and tingling.[65] The majority of the persons were elderly with arteriosclerosis and hypertension. Zeman and Siegel (1947) tested 188 elderly residents in a nursing home.[66] Their final patient was an 83-year-old man who developed a permanent right monoplegia within a few minutes after carotid sinus testing. He had had long-standing hypertension.

On the other hand, many physicians regard the carotid compression test as a safe procedure. Webster and Gurdjian (1958) in their historical review stated, "It has proved to be safe not only in the past but also during present usage in hundreds of patients."[55] Toole and Bevilacqua (1963) reported over 2500 individual vessel compressions with no complications despite the precarious clinical condition of most of the patients.[67] They believed that the diagnostic information gained far outweighs the hazard of the procedure. Between 1963–1977 Fuster (1977) performed without accidents more than 90,000 carotid compressions on more than 12,000 patients.[68] Most persons were between 50 to 85 years of age, many had grossly ulcerated atheromatous plaques or very severe cerebrovascular insufficiency due to stenosis of multiple arterial segments of the carotid and/or vertebrobasilar system, many had cardiac insufficiency or severe arrhythmia, and in 160 patients there was a ruptured intracranial aneurysm with subarachnoid hemorrhage. He stated that the test should be performed only in the laboratory, with appropriate monitoring, and by someone who has mastered the technique and knows how to avoid the risks. It appears to be safer to perform the procedure low in the neck (over the common carotid artery) and not manipulate the carotid bifurcation. Also, it is essential to compress low in the neck in patients who may have an atheromatous plaque from which bits of material could be dislodged.

Like Matas in 1911, Pineda (1966) attempted to enhance collateral circulation by repeated carotid compressions.[69] Patients displaying early signs of cerebral ischemia upon partial or total compression (below a stenosed artery) for very short periods of time were subjected to complete gradual and increasing digital occlusion. When tolerance to occlusion for 2 to 3 minutes was achieved successfully, surgical correction was accomplished. This procedure was said to be useful in performing subsequent carotid endarterectomy without a shunt.

The addition of EEG recording to the carotid compression test increases its sensitivity in the identification of patients with poor collateral circulation. The EEG can indicate brain ischemia before the patient has symptoms. As a result it may reduce compression time and thus reduce the risk of the test. A disadvantage of the compression test, either with or without concomitant EEG, is that it only detects those individuals with an extremely inadequate collateral circulation.[18]

Intraoperative EEG recording during trial clamping of the carotid artery may be used to decide whether or not to use a temporary shunt during endarterectomy. Operating without a shunt may permit better visualization of the posterior wall, a more complete endarterectomy in less time, and more satisfactory placement of intimal tacking sutures when necessary.[70] Insertion of a shunt may cause intimal damage resulting in thrombosis, disruption of the plaque with embolization, or introduction of air into the carotid system. Visualization of the distal end of the plaque may be impaired, especially with a high-lying lesion.[71] Horton and associates (1974) have listed the EEG changes that they believe make the use of an internal shunt mandatory, and point out the additional value to be derived from EEG monitoring in the early recognition and management of intraoperative cerebral embolism or thrombus from an ulcerated carotid lesion.[72]

Published reports show a wide range in percentages of intraoperative

EEG changes. In 399 operations, Callow et al. (1978) stated that 9% showed EEG changes sufficiently severe to require the use of a temporary shunt.[71] Baker et al. (1975) reported that 31 of 157 patients (20%) developed intraoperative EEG changes.[70] Sundt and associates (1974) operated on 113 patients, 25 of whom (22%) developed major ipsilateral EEG changes after carotid clamping.[73] These alterations were reversible following placement of a shunt and reappeared during occlusion for removal of the shunt. Trojaborg and Boysen (1973) reported that 14 of 52 patients (27%) had flattening or slowing of the EEG during two minutes of carotid artery occlusion.[74] Van Gasteren (1979) related that intraoperative EEG changes occurred in 43% of 111 operations.[18,75] This wide variation (from 9% to 43%) may be partially due to lack of uniformity in the definitions of significant and insignificant EEG changes.

Another method of evaluating potential collateral circulation to the brain is by measuring carotid artery backpressure. The first report on intra-arterial blood pressure as measured distal to the temporary clamping site was published by Crawford et al. (1960).[76] They measured pressures ranging from 12 to 90 mm Hg in 17 patients. The highest values were in hypertensive persons with a normal contralateral carotid artery, while the lowest were in those with contralateral occlusion. The authors used temporary internal shunts to protect the brain during carotid endarterectomy, stating that shunts maintained pressures distal to the region of operation essentially equal to those measured in the common carotid artery proximal to the occlusion. Cerebral dysfunction was prevented even though shunts were in use for periods up to 30 minutes.

The term "backpressure" was introduced by Moore and Hall in 1969. They stated:

> We have noticed that the back bleeding from the internal carotid artery in patients who are tolerant of cross clamping is quite brisk, but back bleeding is sparse in patients who are intolerant of carotid cross clamping. This appears to be a qualitative reflection of the adequacy of cerebral collateral circulation. . . . It occurred to us that distal internal carotid artery back pressures could be used to predict tolerance to temporary carotid occlusion.[77]

They observed 48 patients undergoing carotid endarterectomy with local anesthesia. Clamping was not tolerated in 5 persons who had backpressures from 12 to 22 mm HG. The authors stated that clamping appeared safe in patients with backpressures of 25 mm Hg or greater.

Hays and colleagues (1972) defined critical backpressure as 50 mm Hg in a series of 297 operations.[78] Of the 73 operations in which backpressures were less than 50 mm Hg, neurologic deficits appeared postoperatively in 50% of the patients in whom shunts were not used and in 10% of those having shunts. None of the 224 operations done with high backpressures produced strokes. All of their patients had general anesthesia.

The discrepancy between the critical point of Moore and Hall and that of Hays et al. (25 mm Hg vs. 50 mm Hg) may have been explained by Boysen (1973), who stated that elevated intracranial pressure associated with halothane anesthesia was responsible for stump pressures in the 50 to 55 mm Hg range, while the data obtained by Moore and Hall were from patients who were awake.[79]

Since 1977, articles questioning the reliability of backpressure measurements have appeared. Connolly and colleagues (1977) operated on 102 patients under local anesthesia and noted five times that clamping was not tolerated clinically in patients with stump pressures over 25 mm Hg.[18,80] Kwaan et al. correlated the neurologic status of the awake patient with the internal carotid artery stump pressure in 125 persons undergoing carotid endarterectomy.[81] Twenty-four patients lost consciousness immediately after cross clamping, even though stump pressures were above 50 mm Hg in more than one-third of the cases. The majority (80.8%) of the patients tolerated clamping (stump pressures between 20 to 90 mm Hg). This study demonstrated the variability of cerebral tolerance relative to absolute stump pressure guidelines, such as 25 or 50 mm Hg. The authors believed that reliance on these values to determine the need for shunting could lead to a stroke at operation. They stated, "Our experience also showed that assessment of the awake but tranquil patient continues to be the safest and most reliable guide to selective shunting during carotid endarterectomy."[81] Also, a poor correlation between intraoperative EEG recording and stump pressures was found by Brewster et al. (1980).[82] In a series of 80 carotid endarterectomies on 73 patients, 11 of 17 patients with definite ischemic EEG changes had stump pressures greater than 50 mm Hg.

Hertzer et al. (1978) from Cleveland Clinic cited statistics following 260 carotid endarterectomies involving 253 patients.[83] All persons had general anesthesia. The total number of intraoperative deficits was distributed equally among patients with backpressures greater than and less than 50 mm Hg. Eighteen persons had backpressures less than 25 mm Hg and none had intraoperative deficits; 12 of the 18 had shunts and 6 did not. The greatest risk for intraoperative deficits and permanent iatrogenic strokes followed operations done without shunts in the presence of low backpressure. Both high carotid backpressure and the use of shunts in the presence of low backpressure appeared to reduce the risk of permanent strokes. However, the use of shunts in the presence of high back-pressure was associated with an increase in the incidence of neurologic deficits (5), although only 1 persisted as a permanent stroke. Their observations suggest that cerebral embolization during dissection of the carotid artery is a significant factor in the etiology of intraoperative deficits. Ulcerated lesions were present in 92% of patients who developed deficits and in 100% of patients who experienced permanent intraoperative strokes. This appeared to the authors to be more significant than trends of back-pressure and use of shunts.

A fourth method that has been used to evaluate potential collateral circulation to the brain is angiography. Torkildsen and Koppang (1951) first described cross circulation angiographically, although the crossing was already a widely known fact. They reported:

> Valuable prognostic information in cases of contemplated ligation of the internal carotid artery may be obtained by carotid angiography, which readily discloses to what extent one hemisphere may be supplied by arterial blood from the carotid on the opposite side.[84]

Torkildsen and Koppang described four cases showing "collateral circulation that is called into activity when there is partial or complete obstruction of one internal carotid artery."[84]

Mount and Taveras (1957) stated:

> The collateral circulation of the cerebral hemispheres has been clearly demonstrated by cerebral angiography in seriographic films obtained on 42 patients who had had surgical therapy for intracranial aneurysms and on 30 patients who had thrombosis of the internal carotid artery or one of its branches. The potential collateral circulation was found to be very extensive but variable. The first, and most important, source of collateral circulation is through the circle of Willis by way of the anterior and posterior communicating arteries, and, of these, the anterior communicating appears to be the dominant contributor.[85]

In 1960, these same authors wrote that the adequacy of collateral circulation in patients considered for a carotid artery ligation could be determined by carotid angiography. Their criteria for insufficiency of collateral flow were smallness of the divisional part of the contralateral anterior cerebral artery and bilateral demonstration of the posterior cerebral arteries or the filling of both of these vessels when one internal carotid artery was injected and the other was compressed. Bilateral filling of anterior and middle cerebral arteries was an indication of sufficient collateral circulation for ligation of the common carotid, but not for ligation of the internal carotid.[86]

Kirgis et al. (1966) even stated:

> We concluded that because the various patterns of branching of the internal carotid artery can be readily identified by angiography, and since they show a consistent relationship to other segments of the circle, the entire structure of the circle can be predicted quite accurately and its efficiency as a route for collateral blood flow evaluated.[87]

An angiographic test estimating the collateral circulation through the anterior segment of the circle of Willis had already been accomplished on 712 patients by Sedzimir in 1959.[88] After injecting the carotid artery while compressing the opposite carotid, he found that cross-filling through the anterior segment was good in 69%, poor in 24%, and absent in 7% of the patients. There was no difference in these percentages in persons under and over 50 years of age.

Harris and colleagues (1967) compared findings on arteriography with the EEG response to temporary clamping of the carotid artery and found no correlation.[89] Wilkinson et al. (1965) reported a series of 47 patients in which 2 of 3 patients with "exceptionally complete cross-filling" failed to tolerate carotid ligation.[90]

Beatty and Richardson (1968) studied a series of 110 patients undergoing common carotid ligation in a search for clues of prognostic significance regarding postligation cerebral ischemia.[91] Bilateral fetal posterior communicating arteries were associated with a high incidence of intolerance to ligation, but no particular pattern of the circle of Willis was associated with ischemia. They reported:

> Our data indicate that cross-compression studies are of little value in predicting which patients will develop ischemia. The inconsistencies of manual or mechanical artery compression, the relation of the blood pressure to the pressure of injection, and the phase in which the film is taken all make the procedure hard to reproduce. Because of these variables, the amount of cross flow is a difficult criterion to evaluate; it was of no predictive value in this series, a result which is contrary to that of others.[91]

Jawad and colleagues (1977) found that angiography did not provide the important predictive information gained from cerebral blood flow studies.[92] Measuring the regional cerebral blood flow (rCBF) during temporary carotid clamping is another means of assessing the likelihood of a neurologic deficit. The technique of this method will be presented in detail in Chapter 6. In 1966, Jennett et al. reported that rCBF could be measured in the operating room during carotid surgery by the inert-gas-clearance method.[93] The gamma emissions of radioactive xenon-133 are detected through the intact skull after intracarotid injection of a saline solution of the gas. Comparison of the flow before and after temporary clamping of the internal and common carotid artery in turn gives an indication of the risk of cerebral ischemia.

Since 1966, inhaled xenon also has been used to obtain clearance curves to determine cerebral blood flow. The important question has been: how low can the blood flow be reduced in the ipsilateral hemisphere during the 10 to 30 minutes of carotid clamping without damage to the brain?[94] The estimate of the critical level of cerebral blood flow that has to be maintained has varied from 18 ml/100 gm of brain/min. in the studies of Sundt et al. (1974)[73] and Boysen et al. (1974)[94] to 30 ml/100 gm/min. in a report by Prosenz et al. (1974).[95] Permanent ligation of the carotid artery can be performed safely if the cerebral blood flow is more than 40 ml/100 gm/min. (Jawad et al., 1977).[92]

Doppler ultrasound studies can determine the direction of flow in the supraorbital arteries. If used in combination with simultaneous carotid compression, it might estimate the adequacy of the collateral circulation.[18] Kunihiko et al. (1975) compared Doppler signals of a carotid artery before and during compression on the contralateral side.[29] The increase in velocity of flow was seen as a reflection of the adequacy of the collateral circulation. There was a significantly better reaction in young healthy volunteers than in patients with cerebrovascular disease. Bone and co-workers (1977) compared backpressures and direction of supraorbital artery flow during carotid compression.[96] A normal flow direction correlated significantly with higher stump pressures.

Carotid cutaneous photoplethysmography as described by Fuster et al. (1967)[97] and Fuster (1977)[68] records pulses on both earlobes and midfrontal regions. By studying the responses to several carotid compression maneuvers, one can obtain information on the potential collateral supply to the different areas.

Eikelboom (1981) has written a book on the evaluation of carotid artery disease and potential collateral circulation by ocular pneumoplethysmography (OPG) with carotid compression.[18] He performed 1950 tests over a six-year period on patients with symptoms of cerebrovascular insufficiency, patients with asymptomatic bruits, and on persons who had undergone a previous carotid endarterectomy. The opthalmic artery pressure measured on the side of carotid compression was poor (≤60 mm Hg) in about 50% of all tests and good (>60 mm Hg) in 50%. Combined use of preoperative OPG and EEG with carotid compression offers the possibility to select patients who can tolerate intraoperative interruption of the carotid circulation.

Thompson and Talkington (1976) summarized the subject of cerebral ischemia during carotid surgery:

> Neurologic deficits occurring during carotid endarterectomy are caused by cerebral emboli or cerebral ischemia. Although many patients can tolerate temporary clamping of the artery without deleterious effects, the rest require cerebral protection if neurologic deficits are to be avoided. Patients with severe vascular disease and multiple occlusions are least tolerant of clamping.

> Methods presently available to determine the adequacy of collateral blood flow during carotid clamping include temporary occlusion under local anesthesia while checking the neurologic status; determination of stump pressure in the occluded distal internal carotid artery; and EEG monitoring. Although actual determination of the rCBF by the xenon-133 method would be ideal, the technique is rarely available. Clinical investigations indicate that stump pressures of 50–55 mm Hg or higher reflect adequate collateral. . . .

> Present day techniques designed to render cerebral protection during carotid surgery include general anesthesia, induced hypertension, hypercapnia, hypocapnia, temporary intraluminal bypass shunts, and combinations of these.

> General anesthesia is indeed helpful by increasing tolerance of the brain to ischemia and reducing cerebral metabolic demands for oxygen. Induced hypertension is of only moderate benefit in patients with poor collaterals and should not be relied upon; blood pressure should be maintained at or slightly above levels that are normal for the individual patient. Hypercapnia, instead of improving regional perfusion, may result in an "intracerebral steal." Likewise, hypocapnia may be definitely detrimental in areas of focal cerebral ischemia.[98]

They believed that the shunt remains the most reliable method and Thompson used it routinely.

Harris et al. stated, "Regardless of the method used to increase collateral flow in patients with cerebrovascular disease, the results are not always predictable because of anatomic variations of the circle of Willis and alteration of pathways produced by arteriosclerotic lesions."[89]

References

1. Franklin KJ: A Monograph on the Veins. Springfield, IL, Charles C Thomas, 1937.

2. Quiring DP: Collateral Circulation. Philadelphia, Lea & Febiger, 1949.

3. Gurdjian ES, Gurdjian ES: History of occlusive cerebrovascular disease. I. From Wepfer to Moniz. Arch Neurol 36:340–343, 1979.

4. Garrison FH: History of Neurology. Revised and enlarged by McHenry LC, Jr., Springfield, IL, Charles C Thomas, 1969.

5. Heubner D: Die Luetische Erkrankung der Hirnarterien. Vogel, Leipzig, 1874.

6. Fields WS, Bruetman ME, Weibel J: Collateral Circulation of the Brain. Baltimore, Williams and Wilkins, 1965.

7. Van der Eecken HM, Adams RD: The anatomy and functional significance of the meningeal arterial anastomoses of the human brain. J Neuropath Exp Neurol 12:132, 1953.

8. Strandness DE, Jr.: Collateral Circulation in Clinical Surgery. Strandness DE, Jr. (ed), Philadelphia, W.B. Saunders, preface, 1969.

9. Keevil JJ: David Fleming and the operation for ligation of the carotid artery. Brit J Surg 37:92–95, 1949.

10. Abernathy J: Surgical Observations. . . . London, Longmans, pp. 193–209, 1804.

11. Brock L: Astley Cooper and carotid artery ligation. Guy's Hosp Rep 117:219–224, 1968.

12. Willis T: Cerebri Anatome. London, Martin and Allestry, 1664.

13. Willis T: Practice of Physick. London, T. Dring, C. Harper and J. Leigh, 1684.

14. Kramer SP: On the function of the circle of Willis. J Exp Med 15:348–355, 1912.

15. McDonald DA, Potter JM: The distribution of blood to the brain. J Physiol 114:356–371, 1951.

16. Rogers L: The function of the circulus arteriosus of Willis. Brain 70:171–179, 1947.

17. Alksne JF: Collateral circulation. In Collateral Circulation in Clinical Surgery, Strandness DE, Jr. (ed), Philadelphia, W.B. Saunders, pp. 595–609, 1969.

18. Eikelboom BC: Evaluation of Carotid Artery Disease and Potential Collateral Circulation by Ocular Pneumoplethysmography. Utrecht, Uitgeversmaatschappij Huisartsenpers B.V., 1981.

19. Kameyama M, Okinaka S: Collateral circulation of the brain. With special reference to atherosclerosis of the major cervical and cerebral arteries. Neurology 13:279–286, 1963.

20. Alpers BJ, Berry RG: Circle of Willis in cerebral vascular disorders. The anatomical structure. Arch Neurol 8:398–402, 1963.

21. Saphir O: Anomalies of the circle of Willis with resulting encephalomalacia and cerebral hemorrhage. Am J Pathol 11:775–785, 1935.

22. Meyer JS, Fang HC, Denny-Brown D: Polarographic study of cerebral collateral circulation. Arch Neurol Psych 72:296–312, 1954.

23. Leidy J: Abnormal circle of Willis. Trans Path Soc Philadelphia 16:93, 1891–1893.

24. Nishioka H: Report on the cooperative study of intracranial aneurysms and subarachnoid hemorrhage. Results of the treatment of intracranial aneurysms by occlusion of the carotid artery in the neck. J Neurosurg 25:660–682, 1966.

25. Brice JG, Dowsett DJ, Lowe RD: Haemodynamic effects of carotid artery stenosis. Brit Med J 2:1363–1366, 1964.

26. Kelly WA, Strandness DE, Jr.: Anatomy and congenital variations. In Collateral Circulation in Clinical Surgery, Strandness DE, Jr. (ed), Philadelphia, W.B. Saunders, pp. 538–545, 1969.

27. Love JG, Dart LH: Results of carotid ligation with particular reference to intracranial aneurysms. J Neurosurg 27:89–93, 1967.

28. Toole JF: Interarterial shunts in the cerebral circulation. Circulation 33:474–483, 1966.

29. Kunihiko T, Tadaatsu N, Shotaro Y, et al: Assessment of the capacity of cerebral collateral circulation using ultrasonic Doppler technique. J Neurol Neurosurg Psychiat 38:1068–1075, 1975.

30. Meyer JS, Gotoh F, Favale E: Effects of carotid compression on cerebral metabolism and electroencephalogram. Electroencephalogr & Clin Neurophysiol 19:362–376, 1965.

31. Frøvig AG: Bilateral obliteration of the common carotid artery: Thromboangiitis obliterans? Acta Psychiat Neurol Suppl 39:3–79, 1946.

32. Fisher CM: Occlusion of the carotid arteries. Further experiences. Arch Neurol Psych 72:187–204, 1954.

33. Eisenbrey AB, Urrutia AT, Karnosh LJ: Bilateral thrombosis of the internal carotid arteries. Cleveland Clinic Quart 22:174–183, 1955.

34. Batley E: Bilateral internal carotid artery thrombosis. Brit J Radiol 28:472–473, 1955.

35. Clarke E, Harrison CV: Bilateral carotid artery occlusion. Neurology 6:705–715, 1956.

36. Gurdjian ES, Hardy WG, Lindner DW: The surgical considerations of 258 patients with carotid occlusion. Surg Gynec Obstet 110:327–338, 1960.

37. Groch SN, Hurwitz LJ, McDowell F: Bilateral carotid artery occlusive disease. Arch Neurol 2:130–133, 1960.

38. Fields WS, Edwards WH, Crawford ES: Bilateral carotid artery thrombosis. Arch Neurol 4:369–383, 1961.

39. Doniger DE: Bilateral complete carotid and basilar artery occlusion in a patient with minimal deficit. Neurology 13:673–678, 1963.

40. Reuter SR, Newton TH: Bilateral atherosclerotic occlusion of the common carotid arteries. Radiol Clin 33:85–92, 1964.

41. Cravioto H, Rey-Bellet J, Prose PH, et al: Occlusion of the basilar artery. Neurology 8:145–152, 1958.

42. Kingston PN: Case of fatal encephalitis with hemiplegia, immediately excited by cantharides, in consequence of intense predisposition from basilar and internal carotid aneurysms. Edinburgh Med J 57:69, 1842.

43. Hayem MG: Sur la thrombose par arterite du tronc basilaire. Arch de Physiol norm et path 1:270, 1868.

44. Leyden E: Ueber die thrombose der Basilar Arterie. Ztschr klin Med 5:165, 1882.

45. Haugsted H: Occlusion of the basilar artery. Diagnosis by vertebral angiography during life. Neurology 6:823–828, 1956.

46. Lhermitte J, Trelles JO: L'Arterio-Sclerose du Tronc Basilaire et ses Consequences Anatomo-Cliniques. Jahrb Psychiat u Neurol 51:91, 1934.

47. Kubik CS, Adams RD: Occlusion of the basilar artery—a clinical and pathological study. Brain 69:73–121, 1946.

48. Pratt-Thomas HR, Berger KE: Injuries after chiropractic manipulation. JAMA 133:600, 1947.

49. Biemond A: Thrombosis of the basilar artery and the vascularization of the brain stem. Brain 74:300–317, 1951.

50. Freeman I, Ellis WR, Jr., Knox LJ: Occlusion of the basilar artery. An unusual case with recovery. Neurology 3:154–156, 1953.

51. Mount LA, Taveras JM: Ligation of basilar artery in treatment of an aneurysm at the basilar-artery bifurcation. J Neurosurg 19:167–170, 1962.

52. Fields WS, Ratinov G, Weibel J, et al: Survival following basilar artery occlusion. Arch Neurol 15:463–471, 1966.

53. Salomon S: The carotid sinus syndrome. Am J Cardiol 2:342–350, 1958.

54. Crile GW: An Experimental and Clinical Research into Certain Problems Relating to Surgical Operations. Philadelphia, J.B. Lippincott, 1901.

55. Webster JE, Gurdjian ES: Carotid artery compression as employed both in the past and in the present. J Neurosurg 15:372–384, 1958.

56. Calverley JR, Millikan CH: Complications of carotid manipulation. Neurology 11:185–189, 1961.

57. Chevers N: Remarks on the effects of obliteration of the carotid arteries upon the cerebral circulation. London Med Gaz 1:1140–1151, 1845.

58. Parry CH: On the effects of compression of the arteries in various diseases, and particularly in those of the head; with hints towards a new mode of treating nervous disorders. Mem Med Soc London 3:77–113, 1792.

59. Kussmaul A, Tenner A: On the nature and origin of epileptiform convulsions caused by profuse bleeding, and also of those of true epilepsy. London New Sydenham Soc 5:1–109, 1859.

60. Matas R: Testing the efficiency of the collateral circulation as a preliminary to the occlusion of the great surgical arteries. Ann Surg 53:1–43, 1911.

61. Hering HE: Die Karotissinusreflexe auf Herz und Gefässe vom normal–physiologischen, pathologisch–physiologischen und klinischen Standpunkt. Dresden, T. Steinkopff, 1927.

62. Heymans C: Le sinus carotidien et les autres zones vasosensibles réflexogènes. Leur rôle en physiologie, en pharmacologie et en pathologie. London, H.K. Lewis & Co., 1929.

63. Weiss S, Baker JP: The carotid sinus reflex in health and disease. Its role in the causation of fainting and convulsions. Medicine (Baltimore) 12:297–354, 1933.

64. Marmor J, Sapirstein MR: Bilateral thrombosis of anterior cerebral artery

following stimulation of a hyperactive carotid sinus. JAMA 117:1089–1090, 1941.

65. Askey JM: Hemiplegia following carotid sinus stimulation. Am Heart J 31:131–137, 1946.

66. Zeman FD, Siegal S: Monoplegia following carotid sinus pressure in the aged. Am J Med Sci 213:603–607, 1947.

67. Toole JF, Bevilacqua JE: The carotid compression test. Evaluation of the diagnostic reliability and prognostic significance. Neurology 13:601–606, 1963.

68. Fuster B: Carotid cutaneous photoplethysmography test: A method to explore the carotid and vertebral basilar systems. Clin Electroencephal 8:6–26, 1977.

69. Pineda A: Compression of the carotid artery. Evaluation of its prognostic significance before endarterectomy of the carotid artery. Arch Surg 93:415–419, 1966.

70. Baker JD, Gluecklich B, Watson CW, et al: An evaluation of electroencephalographic monitoring for carotid study. Surgery 78:787–794, 1975.

71. Callow AD, Matsumoto G, Baker D: Protection of the high risk carotid endarterectomy patient by continuous electroencephalography. J Cardiovasc Surg 19:55–64, 1978.

72. Horton DA, Fine RD, Lethlean AK, et al: The virtues of continuous EEG monitoring during carotid endarterectomy. Aust N Z J Med 4:32–40, 1974.

73. Sundt TM, Jr., Sharbrough FW, Anderson RE, et al: Cerebral blood flow measurements and electroencephalograms during carotid endarterectomy. J Neurosurg 41:310–319, 1974.

74. Trojaborg W, Boysen G: Relation between EEG, regional cerebral blood flow and internal carotid artery pressure during carotid endarterectomy. Electroencephalogr & Clin Neurophysiol 34:61–69, 1973.

75. Van Gasteren JHM: De endartenectomie van de carotis-bifurcation bij ischemische cerebrovasculaire aandoeningen. Een neurologische retrospectieve en follow-up studie. Thesis, Free University of Amsterdam, 1979.

76. Crawford ES, DeBakey ME, Blaisdell FW, et al: Hemodynamic alterations in patients with cerebral arterial insufficiency before and after operation. Surgery 48:76–94, 1960.

77. Moore WS, Hall AD: Carotid artery back pressure. A test of cerebral tolerance to temporary carotid occlusion. Arch Surg 99:702–710, 1969.

78. Hays RJ, Levinson SA, Wylie EJ: Intraoperative measurement of carotid back pressure as a guide to operative management for carotid endarterectomy. Surgery 72:953–960, 1972.

79. Boysen G: Cerebral hemodynamics in carotid surgery. Acta Neurol Scand 49:suppl 52, 1973.

80. Connolly JE, Kwaan JHM, Stemmer EA: Improved results with carotid endarterectomy. Ann Surg 186:334–342, 1977.

81. Kwaan JHM, Peterson GJ, Connolly JE: Stump pressure. An unreliable guide for shunting during carotid endarterectomy. Arch Surg 115:1083–1085, 1980.

82. Brewster DC, O'Hara PJ, Darling RC, et al: Relationship of intraoperative

EEG monitoring and stump pressure measurements during carotid endarterectomy. Circulation 62 (suppl 1):4–7, 1980.

83. Hertzer NR, Beven EG, Greenstreet RL, et al: Internal carotid back pressure, intraoperative shunting, ulcerated atheromata, and the incidence of stroke during carotid endarterectomy. Surgery 83:306–312, 1978.

84. Torkildsen A, Koppang K: Notes on the collateral cerebral circulation as demonstrated by carotid angiography. J Neurosurg 8:269–278, 1951.

85. Mount LA, Taveras JM: Arteriographic demonstration of the collateral circulation of the cerebral hemispheres. Arch Neurol Psych 78:235–253, 1957.

86. Mount LA, Taveras JM: Further observations of the significance of the collateral circulation of the brain as demonstrated arteriographically. Tr Am Neurol Assoc, pp. 109–113, 1960.

87. Kirgis HD, Fisher WL, Llewellyn RC, et al: Aneurysms of the anterior communicating artery and gross anomalies of the circle of Willis. J Neurosurg 25:73–78, 1966.

88. Sedzimir CB: An angiographic test of collateral circulation through the anterior segment of the circle of Willis. J Neurol Neurosurg Psychiat 22:64–68, 1959.

89. Harris EJ, Brown WH, Pavy RN, et al: Continuous electroencephalographic monitoring during carotid artery endarterectomy. Surgery 62:441–447, 1967.

90. Wilkinson HA, Wright RL, Sweet WH: Correlation of reduction in pressure and angiographic cross-filling with tolerance of carotid occlusion. J Neurosurg 22:241–245, 1965.

91. Beatty RA, Richardson AE: Predicting intolerance to common carotid artery ligation by carotid angiography. J Neurosurg 28:9–13, 1968.

92. Jawad K, Miller JD, Wyper DJ, et al: Measurement of CBF and carotid artery pressure compared with cerebral angiography in assessing collateral blood supply after carotid ligation. J Neurosurg 46:185–196, 1977.

93. Jennett WB, Harper MA, Gillespie FC: Measurement of regional cerebral blood-flow during carotid ligation. Lancet 2:1162–1163, 1966.

94. Boysen G, Engell HC, Pistolese GR, et al: On the critical lower level of cerebral blood flow in man with particular reference to carotid surgery. Circulation 49:1023–1025, 1974.

95. Prosenz P, Heiss WD, Tschabitscher K, et al: The value of regional cerebral blood flow measurements compared to angiography in the assessment of obstructive neck vessel disease. Stroke 5:19–31, 1974.

96. Bone GE, Slaymaker EE, Barnes RW: Noninvasive assessment of collateral blood flow of the cerebral hemisphere by Doppler ultrasound. Surg Gynecol Obstet 145:873–876, 1977.

97. Fuster B, Ferreiro C, Cleaves F, et al: How to explore the patency of the carotid arteries and their collateral circulation by volumetric pulse recordings from both ear lobes. Acta Neurol Latinoamer 13:197–215, 1967.

98. Thompson JE, Talkington CM: Carotid endarterectomy. Ann Surg 184:1–15, 1976.

3

Arteriography

Wilhelm Röntgen.

The discovery of X-rays by Wilhelm Röntgen on November 8, 1895, was acclaimed by the scientific world and also created a sensation in the lay press. Clendening writes that the *Pall Mall Gazette* in January 1896 presented a forthright British judgment on the matter:

> We are sick of the roentgen rays. It is now said, we hope untruly, that Mr. Edison has discovered a substance—tungstate of calcium is its repulsive name—which is potential, whatever that means, to the said rays. The consequence of which appears to be that you can see other people's bones with the naked eye, and also see through eight inches of solid wood. On the revolting indecency of this there is no need to dwell. But what we seriously put before the attention of the Government is that the moment tungstate of calcium comes into anything like general use, it will call for legislative restriction of the severest kind. Perhaps the best thing would be for all civilized nations to combine to burn all works on the roentgen rays, to execute all the discoverers, and to corner all the tungstate in the world and whelm it in the middle of the ocean. Let the fish contemplate each other's bones if they like, but not us.[1]

Even minor poets were inspired, as in this example:

> X-actly So!
> The Roentgen Rays, the Roentgen Rays
> What is this craze?
> The town's ablaze
> With the new phase
> Of X-rays ways.
>
> I'm full of daze
> Shock and amaze;
> For nowadays

>   I hear they'll gaze
>   Thru' cloak and gown—and even stays
>   These naughty, naughty Roentgen Rays.[1]

Nevertheless, the discovery quickly led to a broad investigation of its potential diagnostic value. In fact, only a few weeks after Röntgen's disclosure,[2] a report of the first arteriogram was published by the Austrians Haschek and Lindenthal (1896).[3] Their vascular contrast study was obtained by the instillation of a chalk-containing solution into the arterial system of an amputated upper extremity. The X-ray of the hand appeared in the January 1896 issue of *Wiener klinische Wochenschrift* and clearly showed the potential for visualizing the vascular bed.[4] Although the details were indefinite because of technical limitations, their work must be considered an important milestone in radiographic diagnosis.[5]

However, it was only after the development of suitable contrast media early in the second decade of this century that angiography became practicable on a clinical basis. The discovery of the radiologic value of iodized poppyseed oil (Lipiodol®) was followed by the injection of this material into the antecubital vein of a living human subject by Sicard and Forestier[6] of France (1923), who fluoroscopically followed the progression of the contrast substance through the right cardiac chambers into the pulmonary arteries.[5] The patient coughed as the oil reached the lungs but suffered no other ill effects.[4] The use of strontium bromide and sodium iodide soon followed in efforts to find better and less toxic contrast media.

In 1923, Berberich and Hirsch reported the first brachial arteriogram in man; strontium bromide was the contrast medium. They were studying the physiology and anatomy of the circulatory system.[7] In 1924, Brooks (Figure 3.1) described three cases of femoral arteriography with sodium iodide.[8] He had used this procedure to assist in determining whether a lower extremity should be amputated and, if so, the proper level of amputation (Figure 3.2a,b). Thus, Brooks was the first to report the use of arteriography to determine how a patient should be treated, and so clinical angiography was born.[9]

The first successful opacification of the cerebral circulation in the living human being was reported by Moniz of Lisbon, Portugal (1927), who introduced carotid arteriography (Figure 3.3).[10] He employed direct injection of contrast material into the carotid artery after surgical exposure of the artery. Open methods were used almost exclusively thereafter for the next 10 to 15 years.[11]

Of even greater interest was the demonstration of the feasibility of cath-

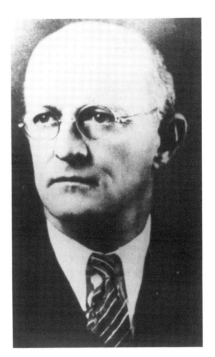

Figure 3.1. BARNEY BROOKS
(From Foster JH: Arteriography: Cornerstone of vascular surgery. Archives
of Surgery 109:605–611, 1974, with
permission from American Medical
Association, Chicago, IL, copyright
1974 and Dr. Foster)

eter angiography by Forssmann, who, in 1929, inserted an oiled ureteral
catheter into one of his own antecubital veins and advanced the catheter
tip into his right heart.[12] His suggestions regarding the injection of opaque
medium through the catheter established him as a pioneer in angiocardiography. Although originally criticized by his colleagues, Forssmann
shared the Nobel Prize in Medicine in 1956 as a result of his original
concept and investigation.[13]

Also in 1929, as related by Abrams,[4] Swick reported the use of an
organic iodide, synthesized by Binz and Rath,[14] known as Selectan.[15] This
drug had been used in the treatment of bovine mastitis and was known
to be excreted in the urine and bile. Because of its iodine content, Swick
thought it might opacify the collecting structures of the kidney during its
excretion following intravenous injection. His supposition proved to be
correct, and this discovery of an opaque organic iodide that was moderately well tolerated when administered intravenously was of immense
importance to the field of angiography.[4,16] When set against the background of rising interest in delineating specific segments of the vascular
bed in man, it proved to be a catalyst of significant proportions. Selectan

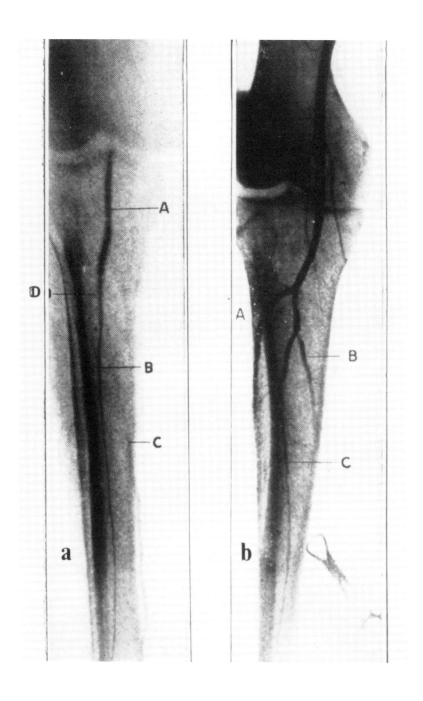

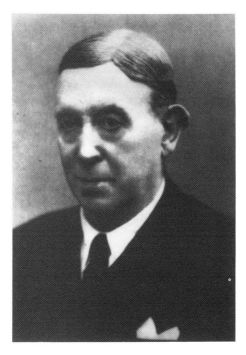

Figure 3.3. EGAS MONIZ
(From Haymaker W, Schiller F: *The Founders of Neurology,* 2nd Edition, 1970. Courtesy of Dr. A. Earl Walker, Albuquerque, NM, and Charles C Thomas, Publisher, Springfield, IL)

Figure 3.2a. Femoral arteriogram by Brooks on September 19, 1923: "(case 1) appearance after intra-arterial injection of sodium iodid: The popliteal (A), peroneal (B) and posterior tibial (C) arteries are injected; there is no injection of the anterior tibial artery; a faint outline of the origin of this vessel can be seen (D). This injection was done without a general anesthetic, and the sharp outlines of the injected vessels are obscured by movement.

Figure 3.2b. "(case 2) appearance after intra-arterial injection of sodium iodid: The popliteal artery shows no obstruction; the anterior (A) and posterior (B) tibial arteries are injected for only a short distance; the lumen of the peroneal artery (C) shows marked irregularities." (From Brooks B: Intra-arterial injection of sodium iodid. JAMA 82:1016–1019, 1924. Courtesy of American Medical Association, Chicago, IL, copyright 1924)

61

was supplemented by Neoselectan (Iopax®) and then by Uroselectan B (Neo-Iopax®). Soon thereafter, Abrodil (Skiodan®) was synthesized, to be replaced by Per-Abrodil (Diodrast®).[4]

Many methods for arteriographic examination of the aorta and great vessels have been developed. Dos Santos, a Portuguese surgeon and urologist (Figure 3.4), and his co-workers reported the first translumbar aortogram in 1929.[17,18] They had often performed translumbar sympathetic blockade with a local anesthetic in patients with peripheral vascular disease. According to Foster (1974), on a number of occasions, the needle was inadvertently inserted into the abdominal aorta.[9] Patients displayed no ill effects after the needle was withdrawn. This observation, coupled with the knowledge of Moniz' work, led them to perform translumbar aortography in man using sodium iodide. In the first few cases, the aortogram was followed by immediate laparotomy to determine whether sub-

Figure 3.4. REYNALDO DOS SANTOS
(From Foster JH: Arteriography: Cornerstone of vascular surgery. Archives of Surgery 109:605–611, 1974, with permission from American Medical Association, Chicago, IL, copyright 1974, and Dr. Foster)

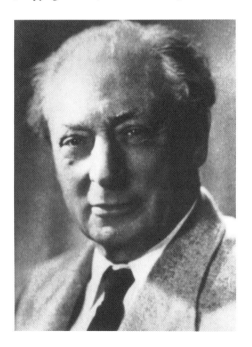

stantial bleeding had occurred. It had not. According to Foster, dos Santos envisioned this technique as more than a means of studying patients with vascular disease. The indications for aortography as recorded in his 1929 report are: gangrene of lower extremities, suppurative osteoarthritis, osteomyelitis, syphilis of bone, Volkmann contracture, sarcomas of bone and soft tissue, and popliteal artery aneurysm. His view was that it would be a valuable method for discovering tumors and other intra-abdominal abnormalities. He also envisioned intra-arterial medications for patients with intra-abdominal infections. Dos Santos termed this aortotherapy. In Paris, in 1931, he reported 300 translumbar aortograms without mortality or appreciable morbidity. These patients, mainly, did not have vascular disease. He was criticized and condemned for doing this reckless procedure without a sound therapeutic indication. Neither dos Santos nor Moniz was interested in vascular disease. Moniz had viewed cerebral arteriograms as a means of demonstrating intracranial tumors. However, their attitudes were understandable—during their time very little could be done about arterial disease.[9]

During succeeding years a number of investigators attempted to opacify the heart in man before Ameuille et al. in 1936 finally succeeded in doing so using the catheter method.[19] A year later the first practical method of angiocardiography was described.[4,20] Also, in 1936, Nuvoli studied the thoracic aorta in man using a percutaneous transthoracic approach, advancing the needle into the thoracic aorta or heart. He delineated aneurysm, tortuosity, and other conditions.[21] Late in 1937, Castellanos (Figure 3.5), Pereiras, and Garcia reported the first successful roentgen contrast diagnosis of a number of congenital cardiac anomalies during life. Between September 1937 and July 1938, they issued many reports; published illustrations of atrial and ventricular septal defects, pulmonic stenosis, the tetralogy of Fallot, and transposition of the great vessels; suggested and performed biplane studies; and devised an automatic injection device which they described in detail.[22–24] One gap in their method of investigating the heart in the living subject was that they were able to opacify adequately only the right heart chambers.[4] Robb and Steinberg in 1938[25] and 1939[26] introduced the use of ether and cyanide circulation times as a guide to the timing of successive exposures in order to obtain sequential opacification of the right and left chambers of the heart. They rapidly injected Diodrast® into an arm vein in 238 patients and made roentgenograms when the chambers of the heart and the great vessels became opaque to the roentgen ray. Robb and Steinberg outlined the four chambers of the heart, pulmonary artery, superior vena cava and its branches, the entire thoracic aorta, and the branches from the aortic arch,

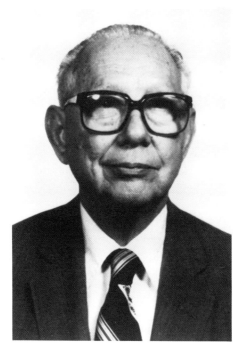

Figure 3.5. AGUSTIN W. CASTELLANOS
(Courtesy of his grandson, Dr. Agustin M. Castellanos)

with no serious consequences. They further suggested the possibility of utilizing cineradiography and rapid serial radiography, as well as coordinating the exposure with the heartbeat.[26] Their technique had three disadvantages: (1) dilution of contrast medium during passage through the cardiopulmonary circuit, (2) difficulty in achieving accurate timing of the arrival of the contrast material in the aorta, and (3) necessity for using a large amount of contrast.[11] Radner is credited with performing the first coronary arteriogram in man (1945).[27] He punctured the aorta through the sternum and injected Thorotrast® (not an organic iodide but an aqueous suspension of a finely particulate thorium dioxide).[28]

The study of the abdominal aorta was dependent on the translumbar approach advocated by dos Santos until 1941, when Fariñas reported the retrograde passage of a urethral catheter into the abdominal aorta through a trocar in the exposed femoral artery.[29] Radner, in 1948, recommended passage of a catheter into the aorta through a "cutdown" on the right radial artery.[30] However, the presence of anatomic anomalies and the frequent occurrence of arterial spasm did not always permit passage of the catheter. Special equipment for injecting the radiopaque material was necessary unless a catheter of large caliber was used, and the method was time-consuming and required radial artery ligation.[11]

The introduction of thin-walled polyethylene tubing, however, made percutaneous catheterization possible, avoiding the time-consuming exposure of an artery and the necessity for sacrificing the vessel after the procedure.[11] In 1953, Seldinger (Figure 3.6), in Stockholm, devised a simple method by which a catheter of the same caliber as the needle could be inserted into the vessel over a flexible wire guide after withdrawing the needle.[31] This innovation completed the groundwork for establishing the modern method of angiography. The catheter method provides a number of advantages: (1) contrast may be injected into a vessel at any level desired, and the circulation of the organ or part under study can be densely

Figure 3.6. SVEN-IVAR SELDINGER
(From American Journal of Roentgenology 142:4, 1984. Courtesy of American Roentgen Ray Society and Williams & Wilkins, Publisher, Baltimore, MD, copyright 1984)

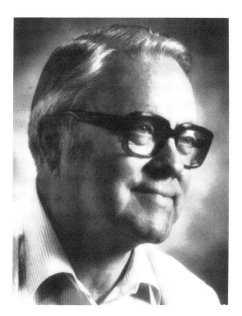

opacified and isolated from the surrounding circulation;[13] (2) the risk of extravascular injection of contrast is minimized; and (3) the patient may be placed in any position necessary to obtain required views.[11] The Seldinger technique truly represented a milestone in the history of angiography. It has been used with millions of patients; countless other investigators have used, refined, and developed his method without need for significant alteration in the basic approach.[32]

Carotid Arteriography

As previously mentioned, Moniz was the first to achieve successful opacification of the cerebral circulation in man (Figure 3.7).[10] He exposed, and temporarily ligated, the internal carotid artery and rapidly injected 30% chemically pure sodium iodide. Roentgenograms of the skull were taken at intervals to demonstrate the opaque substance within the homolateral internal carotid and venous circulation.[33] By 1931 (when his first monograph was published),[34] Moniz had examined 180 patients. Occasionally, sodium iodide caused convulsions or other severe symptoms, and, in 1931, Moniz switched to Thorotrast.[35]

Injection through a direct puncture of the common carotid artery was reported by Loman and Myerson in 1936.[36] They used 5 to 20 cc of Thorotrast in 30 patients with no immediate reactions or late untoward effects. This obviated the need for surgical exposure of the vessel. Turnbull (1939) gave a detailed description of the technique of common carotid puncture and reported 10 cases using this method.[33] It did not receive general acceptance for several years, but after the mid-1940s, it became the one most commonly employed.

Vertebrobasilar Arteriography

Although injection into the internal carotid artery yielded valuable information about the status of intracranial arteries, in most cases only the carotid system was visualized. In his first 600 carotid arteriograms, Moniz noted filling of the vessels in the posterior fossa in only 5 cases.[11] He believed that this occurred because of a reflux of the injected material along the carotid artery to the subclavian, thereby reaching the vertebral. When that happened, it was almost invariably on the right side where the

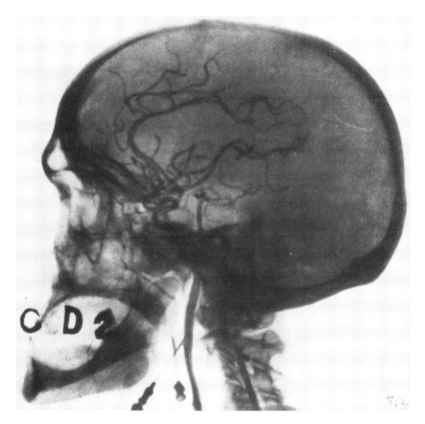

Figure 3.7. Cerebral arteriogram by Moniz, 1927: "Réseau artériel dérivé de la carotide interne. Injection de NaI à 30%" (From Moniz E: L'encéphalographie artérielle, son importance dans la localisation des tumeurs cérébrales. Revue Neurologique 2:72–90, 1927. Courtesy of Masson SA, Paris)

carotid and subclavian arteries originate from a common trunk. In 1933, Moniz, together with his co-workers, Pinto and Alves, reported an open indirect method for injection of contrast into the exposed subclavian artery, making certain the vessel was compressed at a point distal to the vertebral artery.[37] Shimidzu, in 1937, used a closed indirect method with percutaneous injection of contrast into the supraclavicular portion of the subclavian artery while compressing the axillary artery.[38]

Retrograde carotid injection, a technique first reported in 1937 by El-

vidge, has been used fairly extensively.[39] He injected the contrast medium
into the exposed common carotid artery which he compressed distally and
at the same time applied pressure to the axillary artery. Direct injection
into the vertebral arteries has been employed but was fraught with many
complications when one of the Diodrast group of contrast media was used.[11]
Signs and symptoms of brainstem irritation and transient cortical blindness sometimes resulted. Consequently, Thorotrast was used in most of
the early procedures. Berczeller and Kugler, in 1937, suggested an open
direct method which required surgical exposure of the vertebral artery at
the transverse process of the atlas.[40] Lindgren, in 1950, reported 60 cases
in which contrast was injected percutaneously from the front into the vertebral artery at a level high in the neck.[41] In 1938, Sjøqvist described an
open direct method which was a modification of the Moniz technique.[42]
The vertebral artery was exposed close to its origin in the subclavian
artery and Thorotrast was injected directly into it. The closed direct method
for vertebral arteriography was first described in 1940 by Takahashi, who
detailed the anatomic landmarks for determining the point at which the
contrast should be injected percutaneously into this vessel close to its
origin from the subclavian.[43] Unfortunately, none of the methods mentioned thus far were extensively adopted because of the cumbersome technique and lack of reliability of filling with contrast material.

While studying catheter techniques for aortography, Radner noted that
a catheter passed in retrograde fashion through the radial artery had a
marked tendency to enter the vertebral artery. As a result of this observation, he devised the catheter technique of vertebral arteriography, reported in 1947, with which he obtained excellent arteriograms of the vertebrobasilar system.[44] However, it had the disadvantage of requiring ligation
of the exposed radial artery. Gould et al., in 1955, were the first to in-
troduce a method of retrograde injection of contrast medium into the brachial artery by open procedure without using a catheter.[45] Catheter techniques for brachial artery injection were first reported by Sutton[46] and by
Pygott and Hutton[47] in 1959. In 1956, Lindgren described a method for
vertebral artery injection through catheterization of the subclavian from
the femoral artery.[48] This technique was part of his overall project for
selective catheterization of the main trunks originating in the aortic arch.
Interest in the direct percutaneous subclavian puncture, first described by
Shimidzu, was revived in 1957 by Barbieri and Verdecchia.[49] The next
year, in a report concerned with surgical correction of proximal stenosis
and occlusion of the vertebral artery, Crawford et al. recommended a
modification of the Shimidzu method involving direct supraclavicular

subclavian puncture with a Cournand needle in order to visualize the origin of the vertebral artery from the subclavian.[50] For the most part, however, direct supraclavicular subclavian puncture was later abandoned because of the frequency with which the needle penetrated the apex of the pleura, causing pneumothorax. This complication was relatively easily managed but definitely increased the morbidity following the procedure. Pneumothorax became serious if it occurred on both sides following bilateral puncture. In addition, the opacification of the intracranial vessels was frequently of poor quality.

Following this, most investigators adapted the Seldinger technique to axillary artery puncture or infraclavicular subclavian puncture using a double needle with metallic guide for passage of a polyethylene catheter. Direct percutaneous infraclavicular puncture of the subclavian artery was reported by Pouyanne et al. in 1960.[51] In 1964, Weibel and Fields suggested that bilateral simultaneous subclavian injection using a Y-shaped tube would permit more satisfactory delineation of the entire vertebrobasilar arterial system.[52]

Femoral Catheterization

Although many older physicians still use the direct carotid puncture technique which they were taught, most physicians in training today learn the transaortic catheter method via femoral puncture for cerebral angiography. The latter method produces consistently good opacification of carotid and vertebral systems on both sides from their origins upward. Also, using a single catheter and a single femoral artery puncture, the experienced examiner may, in the majority of patients, selectively catheterize any of the major arteries supplying the head and arms. Femoral catheterization may be difficult or impossible in the presence of aortoiliac occlusive disease or extreme tortuosity of the vessels. Attempts to pass a catheter upward in the face of such obstruction may result in dislodging atheromatous plaques and propagation of emboli into the distal vessels of the lower extremities. Furthermore, when the wall of the artery is diseased to the extent that aneurysm formation has taken place, extreme caution must be taken in order to avoid perforating the vessel with the tip of the catheter. The use of a "floppy" wire guide, developed by Rossi in 1966, reduces the possibility of such an occurrence.[53] When femoral catheterization appears impossible or dangerous, the passage of a catheter into the aortic arch can be accomplished by percutaneous puncture of a subclavian, axillary, or carotid artery. The condition of the arteries dictates the choice of the appropriate one.

Digital Subtraction Angiography (DSA)

Subtraction is essentially a method of enhancing the radiographic visualization of contrast media. It was first described by Ziedes des Plantes in 1935, as a photographic method whereby a radiographic negative could be reversed or changed to a positive, after which superimposition of the positive and negative films resulted in the canceling out of identical images on the two films.[54] If one of these films contained added contrast medium, the composite showed only this added material as the prominent feature.[55]

The intravenous injection of contrast medium for the visualization of vascular structures had been introduced by Robb and Steinberg in 1938, but the technique never gained widespread popularity because of the technical problems in obtaining consistently good images. Also, a large amount of contrast material had to be injected to achieve adequate visualization of large arteries, and timing of the circulation was difficult.[56]

Computer technology came to the forefront in the 1970s, and, by the latter part of that decade, reports on computed fluoroscopy (with or without intravenous contrast material) began appearing.[57-59] Digital subtraction angiography combines computer technology with the old radiographic method of intravenous angiography. The images are of moderately good diagnostic quality for visualizing extracranial vessels, and there is lower patient morbidity and mortality as the technique is relatively noninvasive.[56] The quality of the images, both extracranial and intracranial, can be improved with intra-arterial DSA using remarkably small amounts of contrast medium (4 to 8 ml) via femoral artery catheter, and this method also has extremely low morbidity. The procedure can be accomplished on either an inpatient or outpatient basis and is particularly useful clinically for evaluating the extracranial carotid vascular system. DSA is one of the more important radiologic diagnostic advances since computed tomography (CT).[60]

In 1981, Chilcote et al. compared conventional angiography and intravenous DSA for examining the common carotid artery bifurcations in 100 patients with clinically suspected arteriosclerotic disease.[61] In 60% the quality of DSA was good or excellent bilaterally; in 23% the quality was good on one side; in the remaining 17%, both bifurcations were poorly visualized.

Contrast Media

For many years the development of safe and satisfactory contrast media lagged behind the improvement in radiographic equipment and techniques for cannulating or catheterizing specific arteries. From the onset, the toxic potential of sodium iodide was realized. There was local pain and evidence of organic vascular damage. Systemic toxicity of iodism (headache, thirst, feeling of heat, nausea, vomiting, "iodide cold," and fever) was such that the amount of contrast had to be determined with caution. Even death could result from severe iodism.[28] The 1929 discovery of Selectan (5-iodopyridyl-2 sodium oxide) incorporated iodine into an organic radical and thus minimized or eliminated iodism.[28]

There was also a high rate of toxic side effects from Thorotrast and Diodrast. Thorotrast was not metabolized or excreted but was trapped by the phagocytes of the reticuloendothelial system where it caused chronic inflammation and degenerative changes due to its radioactivity.[35] In 1942, a survey of physicians in the United States and Canada by Pendergrass et al. revealed 26 deaths (7 sudden) implicating Diodrast.[62] Four other deaths with Diodrast had been reported previously in the literature and one more occurred at the Hospital of the University of Pennsylvania. This last death prompted the survey.

The introduction of two new groups of water soluble organic iodized preparations was a significant advance in arteriography. The diatrizoate group was made available in the mid-1950s. These agents with or without methylglucamine were much less hazardous and could be used in higher concentrations and smaller amounts while at the same time permitting better visualization than was possible with Diodrast. In 1955, Root and Strittmatter reported the use of new Hypaque® (diatrizoate sodium) in a series of 350 patients.[63] Reactions occurred in 9.7%, mainly nausea, bad taste, vomiting, warmth, and dizziness. It had previously been reported by the Cleveland Clinic that 14.7% of 1000 patients had had reactions from Diodrast.[64] Methyl-glucamine iothalamate was introduced in 1961 and very quickly adopted as the agent of choice by many arteriographers. It could be injected intra-arterially with virtually no discomfort to the patient and minimal signs of vascular or cerebral irritation. It became available in concentrations of 60% (Conray®) and 80% (Angio-Conray®).[11] Bernstein et al.[65] reported their experimental studies with Angio-Conray in 1962, and Weibel et al.[66] published a clinical evaluation of Conray for angiography in patients with cerebrovascular disease in 1963. The latter group used Conray in 192 patients and found little difference between the contrast obtained with it and with Hypaque; side effects with Conray were minimal and transitory even when large amounts were injected during a panarteriographic procedure carried out in one session. Renografin® (sodium methylglucamine diatrizoate) has also been in wide general use for over 30 years.

Experience over this period has proven that these agents are usually safe but may have certain undesirable side effects. These are primarily four types: systemic reactions, cardiac effects, renal effects, and general vascular effects. For the most part, adverse effects are due to combinations of hypertonicity of the ionic contrast agent to blood, calcium binding, and direct chemical toxicity of the specific anion used.[67]

Many attempts have been made to develop new agents, and, in the past six to seven years, nonionic contrast media have undergone extensive experimental evaluation and clinical trial testing.[68–72] These agents have lower tonicity than conventional media at the same iodine content. They also appear to bind calcium less; have less effect on vessel wall, renal function, and hemodynamic and electrocardiographic parameters; and cause less discomfort.[67] It is believed that the pain and feeling of heat often experienced with conventional ionic contrast media are mainly related to their high osmolality compared with that of plasma.[73] The new nonionic media (iohexol, iopamidol) have osmolality approximately twice that of plasma, while ionic agents for angiography have osmolality four (Conray) or five (Renografin) times higher.[67] Also, a small but significant percentage of examinations is degraded by motion artifacts or involuntary swallowing or coughing which are generally attributed to the ionic contrast. New nonionic water-soluble iohexol (Omnipaque®) and iopamidol (Isovue®) reduce these reactions.

Contrast material injected intravenously is used almost routinely in cranial computed tomography to enhance the image of many intracranial lesions, particularly cerebral infarcts. There is little doubt that arteriography will remain as a useful diagnostic tool but it is being used more often now in conjunction with other imaging techniques.

References

1. Clendening L: Behind the Doctor. New York, Alfred A. Knopf, p. 416, 1933.

2. Röntgen WC: On a new kind of rays. Erste Mitt Sitzber Phys-Med Ges (Wurzburg) 137, 1895.

3. Haschek E, Lindenthal OT: A contribution to the practical use of photography according to Röntgen. Wien klin Wochenschr 9:63, 1896.

4. Abrams HL: Introduction and historical notes in Abrams Angiography, Vol. 1, 3rd ed., Abrams HL (ed), Boston, Little, Brown, 1983.

5. Schobinger RA: Milestones in angiography. In Vascular Roentgenology, Schobinger RA, Ruzicka FF, Jr. (eds), New York, Macmillan, 1964.

6. Sicard JA, Forestier G: Injections intravasculaires d'huile iodée sous controle radiologique. C R Soc Biol (Paris) 88:1200, 1923.

7. Berberich J, Hirsch S: Roentgenography of blood vessels. Klin Wochenschr 2:2226–2228, 1923.

8. Brooks B: Intra-arterial injection of sodium iodid. JAMA 82:1016–1019, 1924.

9. Foster JH: Arteriography: Cornerstone of vascular surgery. Arch Surg 109:605–611, 1974.

10. Moniz E: L'encéphalographie artérielle, son importance dans la localisation des tumeurs cérébrales. Rev Neurol 2:72–90, 1927.

11. Weibel J, Fields WS: Atlas of Arteriography in Occlusive Cerebrovascular Disease. Stuttgart, Georg Thieme Verlag, 1969.

12. Forssmann W: Die sondierung des rechten herzens. Klin Wochenschr 8:2085, 1929.

13. Curry JL, Howland WJ: Arteriography Principles and Techniques. Philadelphia, W.B. Saunders, 1966.

14. Binz A, Rath C: Über biochemische eigenschafter von derivaten des pyridins und chinolins. Biochem Z 203:218, 1928.

15. Swick N: Darstellung der niere und harnwege in Röntgenbild durch intravenöse einbringung eines neuen kontraststoffes, des Uroselectans. Klin Wochenschr 8:2087, 1929.

16. Swick N: Intravenous urography by means of Uroselectan. Am J Surg 8:405–414, 1930.

17. dos Santos R, Lamas AC, Pereira-Caldas J: Arteriografia da aorta e dos vasos abdominais. Med Contemp 47:93, 1929.

18. dos Santos R, Lamas AC, Pereira-Caldas J: L'artériographie des membres de l'aorte et ses branches abdominales. Bull Soc Chir Paris 55:587–601, 1929.

19. Ameuille P, Ronneaux G, Hinault V, et al: Remarques sur quelques cas d'arteriographie pulmonaire chez l'homme vivant. Bull Mem Soc Med Hop (Paris) 52:729, 1936.

20. Castellanos A, Pereiras R, Garcia A: La angiocardiografía radioopaca. Arch Soc Estud Clin 31:523, 1937.

21. Nuvoli I: Arteriografia dell'aorta toracica mediante punctura dell'aorta ascendente o del ventricolos. Policlinico 43:227, 1936.

22. Castellanos A, Pereiras R, Garcia A: Angio-cardiographies in newborn. Bol Soc Cuba Pediatr 10:225, 1938.

23. Castellanos A, Pereiras R, Garcia A, et al: On the factors intervening in the obtention of perfect angiocardiograms. Bol Soc Cuba Pediatr 10:217, 1938.

24. Castellanos A, Pereiras R, Vasquez-Paussa A: On a special automatic device for angiocardiography. Bol Soc Cuba Pediatr 10:209, 1938.

25. Robb GP, Steinberg I: A practical method of visualization of chambers of the heart, the pulmonary circulation, and the great blood vessels in man. J Clin Invest 17:507, 1938.

26. Robb GP, Steinberg I: Visualization of the chambers of the heart, the pulmonary circulation and the great blood vessels in man. AJR 41:1–17, 1939.

27. Radner S: An attempt at the roentgenologic visualization of coronary blood vessels in man. Acta Radiol 26:497–502, 1945.

28. Killen DA: Angiographic contrast media: A historical résumé. Surgery 73:333–346, 1973.

29. Fariñas PL: New technique for arteriographic examination of abdominal aorta and its branches. AJR 46:641–645, 1941.

30. Radner S: Thoracal aortography by catheterization from radial artery; preliminary report of a new technique. Acta Radiol 29:178–180, 1948.

31. Seldinger SI: Catheter replacement of the needle in percutaneous arteriography. Acta Radiol 39:368–376, 1953.

32. Dotter CT: Testimonials to Seldinger. AJR 142:8, 1984.

33. Turnbull F: Cerebral angiography by direct injection of the common carotid artery. AJR 41:166–172, 1939.

34. Moniz E: L'angiographie Cérébrale. Paris, Masson, 1931.

35. Sutton D: Arteriography. London, E and S Livingstone, 1962.

36. Loman J, Myerson A: Visualization of the cerebral vessels by direct injection of thorium dioxide (Thorotrast®). AJR 35:188–193, 1936.

37. Moniz E, Pinto A, Alves A: Artériographie du cervelet et des autres organes de la fosse postérieure. Bull Acad Med Paris, 109:758–760, 1933.

38. Shimidzu K: Beiträge zur arteriographie des gehirns—eine einfache percutane methode. Arch klin Chir 188:295–316, 1937.

39. Elvidge AR: The cerebral vessels studied by angiography. A Res Nerv Ment Dis 1:110–149, 1937.

40. Berczeller A, Kugler H: Freilegung der arteria vertebralis am sulcus atlantis. Beitrag zur arteriographie des stromgebietes der arteria vertebralis-basilaris. Arch klin Chir 190:810–815, 1937.

41. Lindgren E: Percutaneous angiography of the vertebral artery. Acta Radiol 33:389–404, 1950.

42. Sjøqvist O: Arteriographische darstellung der gefässe der hinteren schädelgrube. Chirurg 10:377–380, 1938.

43. Takahashi K: Die perkutane arteriographie der arteria vertebralis und ihrer versorgungsgebiete. Arch Psychiat 111:373–379, 1940.

44. Radner S: Intracranial angiography via the vertebral artery. Acta Radiol 28:838–842, 1947.

45. Gould PL, Peyton WT, French LA: Vertebral angiography by retrograde injection of the brachial artery. J Neurosurg 12:369–374, 1955.

46. Sutton D: Vertebral arteriography by percutaneous brachial artery catheterization. Brit J Radiol 32:283, 1959.

47. Pygott F, Hutton CF: Vertebral arteriography by percutaneous brachial artery catheterization. Brit J Radiol 32:114–119, 1959.

48. Lindgren E: Another method of vertebral angiography. Acta Radiol 46:257–261, 1956.

49. Barbieri PL, Verdecchia GC: Vertebral arteriography by percutaneous puncture of the subclavian artery. Acta Radiol 48:444–448, 1957.

50. Crawford ES, DeBakey ME, Fields WS: Roentgenographic diagnosis and surgical treatment of basilar artery insufficiency. JAMA 168:509–514, 1958.

51. Pouyanne A, Caillon F, Leman P, et al: L'angiographie vertebrale par voie sous-clavière sous-claviculaire. Neurochirurgie 3:35–45, 1960.

52. Weibel J, Fields WS: A new technique for craniocervical panarteriography. Acta Neurol Latinoamer 10:60–74, 1964.

53. Rossi P: Transaxillary selective catheterization of the carotid and vertebral arteries. Acta Radiol 5:458–464, 1966.

54. Ziedes des Plantes BG: Eine rontgenographische Methode zur separaten abbildung bestimmter Teile des Objekts. Fortschr Geb Rontgenstrahlen 52:69–79, 1935.

55. Baker HL, Jr.: An assessment of the subtraction technique. Proceedings of Fourth Princeton Conference. In Cerebral Vascular Diseases, Millikan CH, Siekert RG, Whisnant JP (eds), New York, Grune & Stratton, pp. 7–11, 1964.

56. Little JR, Furlan AJ, Modic MT, et al: Intravenous digital subtraction angiography: Application to cerebrovascular surgery. Neurosurg 9:129–136, 1981.

57. Kruger RA, Lancaster J, Mistretta CA, et al: Current results in real time computerized fluoroscopy and radiography. Presented at Work in Progress: Physics session of RSNA, Chicago, Nov 27–Dec 2, 1977.

58. Ovitt TW, Nudelman SN, Fisher D, et al: Computer-assisted video subtraction for intravenous angiography. Presented at Work in Progress: General Diagnosis session of RSNA, Chicago, Nov 27–Dec 2, 1977.

59. Kruger RA, Mistretta CA, Houk TL, et al: Computerized fluoroscopy in real time for noninvasive visualization of the cardiovascular system. Radiology 130:49–57, 1979.

60. Modic MT, Weinstein MA, Chilcote WA, et al: Digital subtraction angiography of the intracranial vascular system: Comparative study in 55 patients. AJR 138:299–306, 1982.

61. Chilcote WA, Modic MT, Pavlicek WA, et al: Digital subtraction angiography of the carotid arteries: A comparative study in 100 patients. Radiology 139:287–295, 1981.

62. Pendergrass EP, Chamberlin GW, Godfrey FW, et al: A survey of deaths and unfavorable sequelae following the administration of contrast media. AJR 48:741–762, 1942.

63. Root JC, Strittmatter WC: Hypaque®, a new urographic contrast medium. AJR 73:768–770, 1955.

64. Mullen WH, Hughes CR: Intravenous urographic contrast media: A controlled trial of Diodrast® and Neo-Iopax®. AJR 68:903–914, 1952.

65. Bernstein EF, Reller CR, Grage TB: Experimental studies of Angio-Conray®; new angiographic agent. Radiology 79:389–394, 1962.

66. Weibel J, Fields WS, Crawford ES, et al: Clinical evaluation of Conray®

for angiography in patients with cerebrovascular disease. AJR 90:1281–1286, 1963.

67. Bettmann MA: Angiographic contrast agents: Conventional and new media compared. AJR 139:787–794, 1982.

68. Sackett JF, Bergsjordet B, Seeger JF, et al: Digital subtraction angiography: Comparison of meglumine-Na diatrizoate with iohexol. Acta Radiol Suppl 366:81–84, 1983.

69. Seeger JF, Carmody RF, Smith JRL, et al: Comparison of iohexol with meglumine-Na diatrizoate for intravenous digital subtraction angiography. Acta Radiol Suppl 366:85–88, 1983.

70. Holtas S: Iohexol in patients with previous adverse reactions to contrast media. Invest Radiol 19:363–365, 1984.

71. Andrew E, Dahlstrom K, Sveen K, et al: Intravascular studies with iohexol (Ominpaque®): Results from first 49 clinical trials. Eur J Radiol 5:68–76, 1985.

72. Dahlstrom K, Shaw DD, Clauss W, et al: Summary of U.S. and European intravascular experience with iohexol based on the clinical trial program. Invest Radiol 20 (suppl 1):117–121, 1985.

73. Dotter CT, Rösch J, Erlandson M, et al: Iopamidol arteriography: Discomfort and pain. Radiology 155:819–821, 1985.

4

Cerebrovascular Surgery

Extensive and sophisticated carotid surgery was performed for aneurysms and for invading cancer many years before its use in the treatment of atherosclerotic disease. The diagnosis was generally obvious in the former cases, whereas carotid occlusion or stenosis could be ascertained in the living patient only after the development of arteriography in the 1920s.[1]

According to Sloan,[2] the first surgeon to restore circulation in the carotid artery after resection was von Parczewski (1916).[3] After removing an arteriovenous aneurysm of the common carotid artery in a 21-year-old male, he performed an end-to-end anastomosis; the patient recovered without neurologic sequelae. Von Haberer (1918) successfully employed resection and lateral suture as well as resection and end-to-end anastomosis in soldiers in World War I.[4] Lexer (1918) recorded a case of traumatic aneurysm involving both the artery and vein in which a resection of 3 cm of the common carotid was made.[5] "During the operation the common carotid was closed for one hour. Paralysis of the opposite leg cleared up the same evening, whereas paralysis of the arm on the same side took four weeks to disappear."[2]

Denk (1918) reported a case of aneurysm of the left common carotid artery in a 20-year-old soldier in whom he united the vessel by a circular suture after the removal of 2 cm of its length.[6] This case was interesting because the author noted the presence of pulsation in the temporal artery after surgery.[2] Sloan's case (1921) was a 56-year-old male with recurrent squamous cell carcinoma of the lower lip and neck. The patient had had previous surgery with much scar tissue, and during dissection the common carotid artery was nicked. The vessel was further damaged by hemostats, and, therefore, that section of the vessel was excised and an end-to-end anastomosis done. The patient recovered without neurologic deficits and had a good temporal pulse.[2]

Conley and Pack (1952) described a novel anastomotic technique used by Conley when it was necessary to excise significant portions of the common and internal carotid arteries because of cancer. An end-to-end anastomosis between the distal stumps of the internal and external carotid arteries allowed "sufficient circulation of blood gained through collateral external carotid branches and the circle of Willis to lessen the hazard of cerebral ischemia and thrombosis in the internal carotid artery and branches, with its attendant disablement or death." The authors also stated, "This anastomosis permits the blood to flow through the anastomotic connections of the external carotid artery from the contralateral side into the external carotid artery of the ipsilateral side and thence into the internal carotid artery and circle of Willis in all instances wherein the arterial blood pressure in the ipsilateral internal carotid artery is less than that in the ipsilateral external carotid artery."[7]

In 1953, Conley reported 11 cases of autogenous vein grafting using the superficial femoral vein or saphenous vein, the first of these operations having been performed in 1951. He wrote, "Autogenous vein graft anastomosis should be considered in every healthy, non-infected neck wound when the treatment of primary tumors such as the carotid body tumors or metastatic tumors in the neck have required excision of the common and internal carotid arteries."[8] Dr. Conley was not a widely known personage in carotid surgery, but as an expert in oncologic surgery of the neck with an impressive series of cases, he was innovative and a true pioneer.[1]

To quote from Foster (1974):

> Prior to the early 1950s, most physicians considered arteriosclerosis to be a generalized systemic disease for which little or nothing could be done. Arteriography was believed to be meddlesome, unwarranted, and dangerous. Following the reports of Oudot[10] (1951) and DuBost and associates[11] (1952) of successful resection and homograft replacement of the abdominal aorta, interest in vascular surgery skyrocketed. It soon became apparent that, while arteriosclerosis is a generalized disease, it also is often characterized by short, segmental occlusive lesions amenable to surgical correction.[9]

Although, as mentioned in Chapter 1, Penzoldt (1881) had described thrombosis of the common carotid artery, and Chiari (1905) and Hunt (1914) had emphasized the importance of extracranial carotid disease, the condition received little attention. Routine postmortem examination seldom included study of the cervical vessels, and arteriography was considered too hazardous for elderly persons with arteriosclerosis. Binswanger and Schazel (1917)[12] suggested that chronic progressive subcortical encephalitis was due to atherosclerosis, and, in 1925, Dow[13] reported that the carotid bifurcation and carotid siphon are sites of predilection for atheromatous changes and occlusion. Hypertensive encephalopathy was described by Oppenheimer and Fishberg[14] in 1928, while Spielmeyer (1928)[15] was among the first to recognize the effects of transient cerebrovascular insufficiency.

Early modern scientific study of cerebral arteriosclerosis was described by Wolkoff (1933),[16] and, in that same year, Keele[17] reported a study of 55 consecutive autopsies showing atheromatous changes in the carotid sinus in 50 cases. The first report of internal carotid thrombosis demonstrated by cerebral angiography was that of Sjøqvist in 1936.[18] The occlusion was just above the carotid siphon, and a presumptive diagnosis of a thrombosed aneurysm was made.[19] The following year, Moniz, Lima, and de Lacerda described occlusion of the cervical portion of the internal carotid artery.[20] Their report included clinical details of four cases in which the diagnosis was made by arteriography. They believed that thrombosis must frequently take place with few or no symptoms, for surgical ligation of the internal carotid artery could be carried out in many cases without sequelae.

In 1935, Leriche and colleagues recommended resection of the entire occluded artery, but this was not technically easy to perform.[21] In 1938, Chao et al. in Peiping, China, described operations of two cases of left internal carotid thrombosis.[22] The first patient had transient ischemic attacks (TIAs) with gross difficulty in word finding, memory, and calculation. Following an arteriogram (with thorium dioxide) which showed occlusion of the internal carotid artery, an arterectomy was done. The authors did not intend this as treatment; it was to substantiate the diagnosis. After the operation, they stated that the patient improved mentally. The second patient had suffered a major stroke 13 months prior to their examination. He had deficits of right hemiplegia, hemianopia, and aphasia. The left internal carotid artery was occluded. Surgery was for treatment: denervation of an abnormally reacting carotid sinus and excision of a thrombosed carotid artery. The patient had hypertension and signs of considerable brain damage. Their idea was to prevent cerebral ischemia by relieving irregular hypertension due to a hypersensitive carotid sinus. The removal of the thrombosed segment interrupted the continuity of sympathetic impulses in the walls of the artery.

In addition to these clinical reports, Hultquist, in 1942, published his extensive monograph describing the results of the pathological study of the entire carotid system in a series of 1400 autopsies.[23] He studied the location, pathogenesis, histology, and propagation of thromboembolism, giving detailed accounts of the resultant changes in the brain. However, little or no attempt was made to correlate clinical data with anatomical findings.[24]

In 1951, Johnson and Walker reported that routine angiography in 500 patients revealed 6 to have complete carotid occlusion.[19] They noted that 101 cases had been mentioned previously in the literature, 84 being European and only 17 American. Johnson and Walker suggested, as did Fisher that same year, that carotid occlusion probably is far more frequent than had been reported.[24] It was believed that the presence of a thrombosed vessel might result in a reflex spasm of the smaller cerebral vessels, and was suggested that this might account for the transient nature of some symptoms.[19]

The etiology of carotid thrombosis was unknown in 1951. Johnson and Walker reported that syphilis probably played little role—only 2 cases of the 107 reported until then had positive serologic reaction. The blood pressure had usually been normal and in only 10 cases was it over 180 mm Hg. In 13 cases there was history of head trauma. Several authors suggested retrograde thrombosis from an intracranial aneurysm or retrograde extension of a thrombus originating in a cerebral vessel. In none of the cases where autopsy was performed was this hypothesis confirmed. The two most common factors appeared to be arteriosclerosis and thromboangiitis obliterans.[19]

Fisher's report in 1951 is considered to be a truly landmark article (Figure 4.1). He presented eight cases, emphasizing the relation between obstruction of carotid arteries in the neck and cerebrovascular insufficiency and stated that thrombosis of the internal carotid artery is much more frequent than suspected and might prove to be a major cause of apoplexy.[24]

All of Fisher's cases, except one, had prodromal fleeting symptoms of paralysis, numbness, tingling, aphasia, unilateral blindness, or dizziness. However, he stated that the fundamental disturbance underlying TIAs was unknown.

The fact that carotid thrombosis often takes place with few or no symptoms and that the extent of the damage to the brain following spontaneous occlusion of an internal carotid artery is a function of the adequacy of the collateral circulation were also mentioned by Fisher. He believed the recognition that carotid occlusion takes place as a result of local arterial disease had long been delayed. Fisher stated:

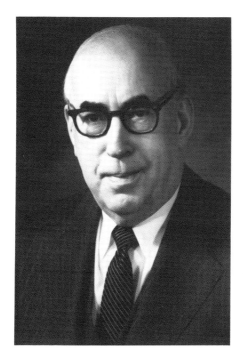

Figure 4.1. C. MILLER FISHER

. . . the frequency with which coronary atherosclerosis, cardiac infarction, angina pectoris, peripheral gangrene, intermittent claudication, and absence of pulse at the ankle accompany disease of the internal carotid artery is in keeping with the generally accepted idea that the process is atherosclerotic.[24]

Fisher expressed his belief that unexplained cerebral embolism may arise from thrombotic material lying in the carotid sinus and predicted:

. . . it is conceivable that some day vascular surgery will find a way to by-pass the occluded portion of the internal carotid artery during the period of ominous fleeting symptoms.[24]

Also in 1951, Fisher and Adams wrote:

. . . nearly all cases of hemorrhagic brain infarction are of embolic origin. The blockage of an artery by an embolus causes infarction of the tissue supplied by that vessel. Later, due to fragmentation of the embolic material and possibly to relaxation of local vascular spasm, the embolus moves from its original position into more distal branches. This exposes the necrotic tissue to the full force of arterial blood pressure with resulting hemorrhages from damaged capillaries.[25]

In 1954, Fisher reported:

> Mural thrombus deposited upon atherosclerotic ulceration within the carotid sinus is not infrequent, especially if smaller microscopic deposits are included. Small emboli must often break away without causing symptoms, or even cerebral lesions. . . . It has not been possible to get a clear understanding of the manner in which such emboli arise. Slowing of the blood flow, turbulence, or mural deposits are among the possibilities. In one case, the embolic material was wholly composed of platelets.[26]

To our knowledge, Gordon Murray performed the first successful surgery to restore circulation in an occluded common carotid artery on September 20, 1950, in Toronto.[1,27] The patient was a 54-year-old white male with syphilitic aortitis and obliteration of all four great vessels. He had had about 14 generalized convulsions during the four years before admission. No pulses could be obtained in any of the arteries of the arms or neck. Blood pressure could not be ascertained in either arm. Retrograde aortograms via the femoral artery revealed normal aortic caliber with a small saccular aneurysm at the arch. "The left common carotid artery was opened and found to have a patent though contracted lumen. A probe was passed down through the vessel until firm resistance was encountered at the place where the vessel arose from the aorta. The probe was passed into the aortic lumen, and a free flow of blood returned into the carotid. The opening was enlarged by further instrumentation until a very good pulsatile flow came into the carotid. The carotid artery was closed and good pulsation was felt in the vessel above the operative site."[27]

On October 20, 1951, Carrea, Molins, and Murphy of Buenos Aires operated a patient with spontaneous thrombosis of the cervical internal carotid artery. They had previously operated two other patients, in one resection of the carotid bifurcation was performed, and, in the second, extirpation of the diseased internal carotid artery (cervical sympathectomy was included in both cases). The third case was reported by them in greater detail. That patient, a 41-year-old wealthy wine merchant from Mendoza, Argentina, was first seen by the neurologist Guillermo Murphy because of sudden loss of consciousness, right-sided jacksonian seizures, right hemiplegia, and loss of sight in the left eye. He was also noted to have evidence of atherosclerosis of the lower limb arteries. Murphy had just received his copy of the *Archives of Neurology and Psychiatry*, in which Fisher had described cerebral symptoms associated with internal carotid artery occlusion. Murphy believed that the patient's symptoms which were precipitated by gastrointestinal hemorrhage, resulting in acute anemia, were consistent with Fisher's description. The patient was persuaded to accompany Murphy to Buenos Aires to see Raúl Carrea (Figure 4.2), a neurosurgeon who had only recently returned to Argentina from the Neurological Institute of New York. Carrea performed left percutaneous carotid angiography, which showed severe stenosis of the internal carotid about 12 mm above the bifurcation. Mahels Molins, a thoracic surgeon, assisted him in the subsequent operation. In this case, following cervical sympathectomy and ligation of collaterals of the external carotid artery, the internal carotid was cut above the abnormal area and the external carotid was also cut at the same level. The proximal portion of the external carotid was anastomosed end-to-end to the distal portion of the internal carotid. The atherosclerotic plaque of the internal carotid was partially ablated and the lumen of the artery was entirely occluded at its origin with ligatures. On the 15th postoperative day, a carotid angiogram

Figure 4.2. RAÚL CARREA
(Courtesy of Dr. Ramón Leiguarda, Buenos Aires)

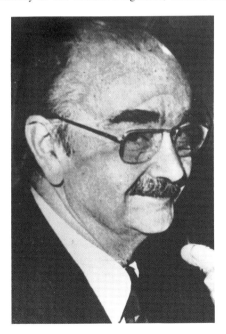

showed that "the common carotid suddenly narrowed to continue with a carotid vessel of regular diameter and smooth walls where it was difficult to ascertain the location of the suture." The anterior and middle cerebral arteries were normally filled. On discharge, the patient's gait was almost normal and "hardly any difference could be noticed between the reflexes of both sides." Loss of sight in the left eye remained unchanged.[28]

Thromboendarterectomy

By the late 1940s, medical journals in France began featuring accounts of a new procedure named "thromboendarterectomy," which resulted in improved circulation in arteriosclerotic peripheral vessels or in the aorta.[29-34] The operation, first performed by Jean Cid dos Santos, consists of resection of the intima and diseased portion of the media together with the thrombus.[29] It depends on the existence of a pathologic cleavage plane within the media. It is in this plane that the accumulation of cholesterol, fatty acid salts, and tissue debris creates a line of separation between the relatively uninvolved outer coat and the diseased intima of the artery.[35] In the United States, Wylie et al. (1951)[35] described their experiences with the use of fascia lata applied as a graft around arteries after thromboendarterectomy, and, in 1952, Wylie published case histories of thromboendarterectomy for peripheral arteries.[36]

The first thromboendarterectomy for occlusion of the internal carotid artery in the neck was probably performed by Hurwitt on January 28, 1953, as reported by Strully, Hurwitt, and Blankenburg. The patient had suffered a major stroke 16 days before surgery and the lesion was diagnosed and verified by angiography (Diodrast). At operation, a 7 cm piece of clot was removed, but the distal part of the clot could not be completely extricated. The artery was ligated and a 2 cm portion resected because of the danger of dislodging the clot into the intracranial portion of the artery when the clamp on the common carotid artery was removed.[37]

In 1975, DeBakey reported that he had operated on a patient on August 7, 1953, and he believed this to be the first successful thromboendarterectomy for cerebrovascular insufficiency caused by atherosclerotic occlusion of the carotid artery, as well as the longest follow-up study. At the time of the patient's death from coronary occlusion 19 years after operation, he had no cerebrovascular symptoms and there was clinical evidence of maintenance of the restored circulation in the carotid artery.[38]

However, at the time, the most noteworthy and widely publicized reconstruction of a thrombosed carotid artery was that of Eastcott, Pickering, and Rob reported in 1954.[39] They stated that previous surgical treatment had been along three lines: arterectomy (Chao et al.) in the hope that removal of the diseased segment might reduce reflex spasm in the cerebral vessels; cervical sympathectomy (Johnson and Walker) with the same objective; and thromboendarterectomy (Strully et al.). Eastcott et al. believed that all these procedures were ineffective. They described a case in which a partially thrombosed segment of the common and internal carotid arteries was resected and the blood vessel reconstructed by a direct anastomosis. The patient had had a total of 33 TIAs and further episodes were prevented by the surgery. The patient also had had attacks strongly suggesting paroxysmal tachycardia. The authors reported:

> It is well recognized that paroxysmal tachycardia may cause faintness and even loss of consciousness, and in the presence of a gross obstruction of the internal carotid artery, such as was found here, ischemic symptoms in the territory supplied would not be surprising.[39]

The patient had had an arteriogram by direct puncture of the left carotid. That surgery (Figure 4.3) set the stage for and was the herald of contemporary carotid surgery.

In a recent (August 1987) letter to the authors, Mr. Eastcott (Figure 4.4) recalls that event:

> The operation on May 19th 1953 was photographed by a visiting surgeon, a member of a distinguished Travelling Club from the States which included Drs. DeBakey and Wylie, to whom Charles Rob showed the patient on their Ward visit the previous day. He remembers that Jack Wylie suggested that an endarterectomy should be considered. In the event, I was given the freedom to make my own operative decision, in the generous and wise way that Charles has with his juniors, and I elected to excise the bifurcation and anastomose the common and internal carotid arteries, just as I had so often done in my Harvard Medical School days, and in an old man with malignant lymph nodes involving the common carotid, about a year before the present case. It took 28 minutes of clamp time, the cerebral protection being provided by induced hypothermia at 28 C. The photographer that day was none other than Dr. George Dunlop, who many years later in 1977, as President of the American College of Surgeons, invested me as Honorary Fellow!
>
> He lent the slide to Dr. Jesse Thompson for his lecture to the Society of Vascular Surgeons/International Cardiovascular Society, at Albuquerque in 1976 (I believe it was), at which Jesse made a most glowing reference to our influence in setting this whole surgical activity into motion. It came

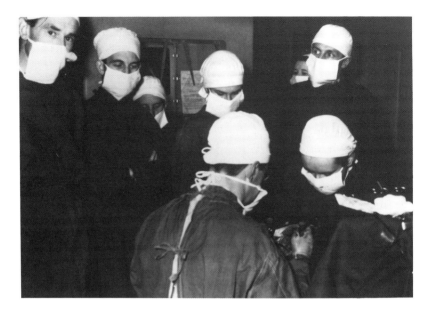

Figure 4.3. The landmark carotid reconstruction operation at St. Mary's Hospital, London, May 19, 1953, with Mr. H. H. G. Eastcott (back to camera) operating and Mr. Charles Rob (standing) in left corner of picture. (Courtesy of George R. Dunlop, M.D., Worcester, MA)

> as a total surprise to me at the time, for I never knew that any photograph had been taken. (personal communication)

It appears that Edwards and Rob (1956) published the first report of complete recovery from a reversible ischemic neurologic deficit (RIND) following surgical therapy.[40] Their patient, with a partial (80%) occlusion of the left internal carotid artery, was unable to sign his name, had slurred speech, and abnormal pyramidal signs and symptoms in his right upper and lower limbs. These abnormalities had been present for eight weeks. Following resection of the diseased segment of the artery and direct anastomosis of the common and internal carotid arteries, the patient awoke to find his deficits completely cleared. "And his pleasure at this, plus the usual euphoria seen after operations under hypothermia, produced an elation which can seldom have been equalled."[40]

The first documented use of a temporary shunt during carotid endarterectomy was that by Cooley et al. on March 4, 1956. They described:

A polyvinyl shunt, with needle points at both ends, was used to by-pass the carotid circulation during the period of occlusion. With the external carotid temporarily occluded, internal carotid flow was maintained by means of the shunt while the atheromatous plaque was removed from the vessel. The intervening segment of artery was occluded by arterial clamps and a transverse incision was made in the arterial bulb. The occluding calcified arteriosclerotic plaque was peeled out of the lumen by thromboendarterectomy and the arteriotomy was sutured transversely. Arterial flow was restored after 9 minutes of carotid clamping during which period the shunt continued to function satisfactorily.[41]

They used large bore needles (14 to 16 gauge) at the ends of the shunt.

In 1958, Fields, Crawford, and DeBakey documented replacement of vessels with dacron.[42] Bypass grafts using a specially designed flexible dacron tube were employed in patients with extensive occlusions of the innominate and carotid arteries.

The first vertebral artery ligation may have been by Maisonneuve and

Figure 4.4. H. H. G. EASTCOTT

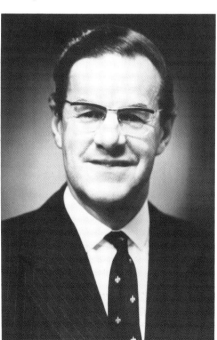

Favrot in 1852, performed for a gunshot wound. This information was related by Rudolph Matas during a discussion of vertebral ligation.[43]

In 1956 and 1957, Hutchinson and Yates reported on anatomic studies in patients dying of cerebrovascular accidents.[44,45] The vertebral arteries were involved with occlusive lesions in approximately 39% of cases. They stated:

> Another aspect of vertebral-artery stenosis, and one of some importance, is that such stenosis alone may be responsible for infarction of the brain without either occlusion of the intracranial vessels or disease of the carotid arteries.[45]

In 1958, Crawford, DeBakey and Fields reported techniques for endarterectomy and bypass of obstructed vertebral vessels. They related:

> Atheromatous occlusions of the internal carotid artery in the neck and the great vessels at their origins from the aortic arch have emerged as clinical entities characterized by manifestations of arterial insufficiency in the distribution of the anterior and middle cerebral arteries. The frequent discrete and localized nature of the occlusive process in such patients has led to the application of reconstructive arterial techniques designed to restore normal cerebral circulation. A large number of patients have now been successfully treated with these techniques . . . studies of Hutchinson and Yates showed that the vertebral arteries may be similarly involved. . . . The clinical significance of this finding is obvious, and the extracranial location of these lesions suggests the possibility of direct surgical attack.[46]

They described their surgery on 43 lesions in the internal carotid, innominate, subclavian, and left common carotid arteries. They believed that persistent neurologic deficits including weakness, aphasia, visual disturbances, and mental obtundity, which occurred before operation, had been relieved. They used percutaneous injections of Hypaque into the subclavian artery for angiography.

Also in 1958, Fields et al. stated:

> The lesion causing cerebral arterial insufficiency is located outside the skull in approximately 25% of patients with stroke syndromes. . . . A definite diagnosis is possible only by angiography.[42]

In 1959, Cate and Scott described their first subclavian-vertebral artery thromboendarterectomy.[47] The patient was first seen in June 1957. He had a weak, cold left upper extremity with absent pulse, unsteady gait, dizziness, and headache. They believed that the arm symptoms were not sufficient to justify major surgery, especially in view of cerebral disease.

They concluded that diffuse intracranial arterial occlusion was the source of the cerebral symptoms.

However, after reading the Hutchinson and Yates publication, they became aware of the importance of the vertebral arteries in the cerebral circulation. On September 7, 1957, combined subclavian-vertebral thromboendarterectomy was done. They had used a catheter via the femoral artery and injected Hypaque for arteriography. After operation, the blood pressure was equal and normal in both arms, and the patient's symptoms cleared. He went back to work.

Joint Study of Extracranial Arterial Occlusion

By the late 1950s, it had become apparent that the improvement of contrast media over the previous decade and the development of reconstructive arterial surgery for the treatment of occlusive disease had brought about a change in the approach to the stroke patient. Carotid endarterectomy was becoming commonplace worldwide. In January 1959, plans were formulated by a group under the direction of Dr. Michael E. DeBakey (Figure 4.5) for a cooperative study to determine the efficacy of such surgery and to compare it with the customary medical treatment. The study, supported by the National Heart Institute in Bethesda, was officially designated the Joint Study of Extracranial Arterial Occlusion. Initially, there were 10 participating institutions in the United States; this number gradually increased to 24, including one center in Montevideo, Uruguay.

This trial provided the opportunity to characterize, both clinically and angiographically, a large group of patients with cerebrovascular disease and to observe in detail their long-term clinical course. Between July 1959 and July 1970, information was recorded on a total of 6535 patients (69% men, 31% women). Soon after the inception of the Joint Study, it became evident that the determination of the efficacy of surgery in modifying the course of cerebrovascular disease required a controlled trial. In 1961, 5, and later 13, of the 24 institutions agreed to assign patients for surgery at random, using common criteria. This was the first trial in the United States in which large numbers of patients were randomly allocated to surgical or nonsurgical therapy.

As the Joint Study evolved, valuable data on many aspects of cerebrovascular disease were accumulated. This "spin-off" information provided the source material for numerous articles. Between 1968 and 1976, 10 official reports were published in the *Journal of the American Medical*

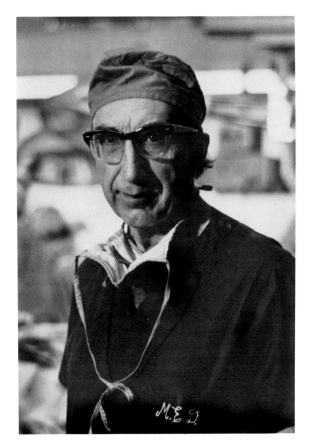

Figure 4.5. MICHAEL E. DEBAKEY

Association,[48–57] but many other articles based on Joint Study statistics have appeared in other periodicals.

Review of the randomized series showed no significant difference in long-term survival between the medical and surgical groups. Beneficial effects of surgery could not be substantiated when death was selected as the endpoint. Analysis of mortality data showed that the most common cause of death in patients with ischemic cerebrovascular problems was cardiac disease. During the relatively short follow-up period (average three years), any potential benefit from surgical prevention of stroke was obscured by the high immediate postsurgical mortality. This made comparison of the medical and surgical groups for the true incidence of stroke virtually impossible.[58]

In the first years of the Joint Study, surgical mortality was high, presumably because of inexperience with the technical aspects of the operation and often inappropriate selection of patients for surgery. In the first five years of the Joint Study, for example, patients were operated as early as possible after the onset of an acute neurologic deficit in an effort to reverse the damage. It was soon realized that mortality was twice as high in the surgical group as in the medical cohort—probably because of the conversion in the former of ischemic infarcts into the far more lethal hemorrhagic infarcts.[59,60] This overshadowed any potential long-term benefit from decreasing morbidity from stroke.[51]

When the participants of the Joint Study agreed to common indications to qualify for surgery in 1961, the etiology of stroke was believed to be related to altered blood flow and cerebral perfusion; a lesion was not considered significant unless it was obstructing flow. Thus, many patients with nonobstructing, ulcerated plaques were excluded from randomization and from surgery. As the Joint Study progressed, it was recognized that embolism from an atherosclerotic plaque might be more important than obstruction as a pathogenetic factor, but surgical indications were not redefined, since it was necessary to keep the series consistent to permit pooling of the collected data.[58] There was a progressive decrease, however, in operative mortality in unilateral carotid bifurcation operations from 9.5% in 1961 to 2.8% in 1969.

Also, patients with cardiac disease had a significantly higher mortality when treated surgically, as opposed to medically. Among those patients, it was likely that disability and death would be caused by cardiac problems, and the risk of operation and attendant postoperative complications were higher. The risk was also increased by the presence of concurrent hypertension or diabetes.

Although the evidence obtained from the Joint Study had many shortcomings and was inconclusive, it was recently reviewed by Warlow, who stated, "the fact that the trial was done at all remains a remarkable achievement, particularly when one remembers that at the time the climate of opinion towards randomised trials was not so favorable as it is today."[61]

In addition to comparing surgical and medical management of patients with ischemic cerebrovascular disease, reports from the Joint Study data: (1) produced detailed demographic information based on 6535 patients; (2) described arteriographic techniques, sites, and complications; (3) delineated racial differences in the clinical and arteriographic manifestations of stroke; (4) confirmed risk factors for stroke; (5) reported the frequency, distribution, and types of atherosclerotic lesions; and (6) gave specific accounts of various subgroups of patients, i.e., those having transient ischemic attacks, subclavian steal syndrome, and internal carotid artery occlusion.

Until 1984, the report from the Joint Study (1969) was, to our knowledge, the only publication in the world describing a controlled randomized trial of carotid endarterectomy. The primary result of the Joint Study, namely, that there was no statistically significant difference in stroke or death outcomes between the surgical and medical groups, has been forgotten over the years. It has been overshadowed by the enthusiasm of surgeons and by reports of nonrandomized surgical series citing good results.

In 1984, Shaw et al. reported a small study with 20 patients randomly allocated to surgery, 21 no surgery.[62] The results were consistent with those of the Joint Study and did not show an overall benefit for carotid endarterectomy compared with medical treatment.

A controlled trial of carotid endarterectomy in men who have been determined to have asymptomatic carotid stenosis has been conducted under the auspices of the United States Veterans Administration since 1982. Enrollment has been completed and the patients are being followed prospectively. At present, a randomized trial of carotid endarterectomy is also under way in the United Kingdom, France, Holland, Germany, and Italy. Two others, one in persons with asymptomatic carotid stenosis and the second in patients with carotid lesions and transient ischemic attacks or minor stroke, have been funded by the National Institutes of Health in Bethesda and have begun recruiting subjects.

Gradually, carotid endarterectomy has become one of the most commonly performed operations in the United States and Canada, and, in recent years, the appropriateness of this conspicuous increase has come under attack. Data from the National Hospital Discharge Survey, the Veterans Administration Hospitals, and Armed Forces Hospitals indicate that the number of endarterectomies of extracranial vessels of the head and neck performed in the United States increased from around 15,000 in 1971 to around 85,000 in 1982[63] and to 103,000 in 1984.[64] An estimated 2.8% of those operated in nonfederal hospitals were discharged dead.[63] It has been estimated that there are only approximately 35,000 patients each year who have appropriate symptomatic angiographic lesions.[65] If this figure is correct, there are thousands of persons operated each year under circumstances that many physicians would question. The incidence of stroke or death caused by endarterectomy varies widely among surgical series; a recent review of 18 series showed a risk ranging from 2.5% to 24.4%.[61]

It is an indisputable fact that innumerable patients have benefited from endarterectomy and no physician would refuse to consider surgery for a symptomatic person who has a flow-obstructing or ulcerated lesion at the bifurcation. Concern arises over the sizable number of operations on asymptomatic individuals who may have midcervical bruits or smooth stenotic lesions not large enough to affect blood flow. Some physicians believe that many persons in the United States have undergone carotid endarterectomy unnecessarily. If such is the case, perhaps the widespread publicity recently bestowed on this situation will induce some surgeons to consider changes in their criteria for selection of eligible patients.

Subclavian Steal Syndrome

In 1960, Contorni reported visualization of the vertebral and subclavian arteries on one side following injection of contrast medium into the opposite subclavian artery.[66] In January 1961, at the Third Princeton Conference on Cerebrovascular Diseases, Toole (during a discussion on arteriography) mentioned that he had encountered two patients with stenosis of the left subclavian artery just distal to its origin, in whom there was retrograde filling of the left vertebral artery, from the basilar artery toward the left subclavian.[67] In other words, flow was reversed in the vertebral artery. He stressed that if arteriography by direct vertebral puncture had been performed, only vessel patency would have been shown and not the important pathophysiology, i.e., reversal of flow. One patient had symptoms of basilar artery insufficiency, but the second patient did not.

At the same meeting, Rob stated:

> In one of our patients the blood supply of the brain was actually improved by ligature of an extracranial cerebral artery. This patient, a left-handed man, had an occlusion of the first part of the right subclavian artery, no abnormality was noted in either the carotid or vertebral arteries apart from the fact that contrast medium injected into the left vertebral artery rapidly appeared in the right vertebral artery. It was our opinion that the transient attacks of cerebral ischemia in this patient were due to blood being withdrawn from the cerebral circulation into the right arm when that limb was exercised. Ligature of the right vertebral artery just distal to the complete right subclavian occlusion stopped the transient attacks of cerebral ischemia in this patient.[68]

In November 1961, Reivich and associates published a report of two patients in whom they observed retrograde blood flow in the left subclavian artery. They wrote:

> In both cases the anatomic lesion producing the reversal of blood flow was a stenosis of the left subclavian artery proximal to the origin of the vertebral artery. The cause of the reversed flow in these circumstances can be attributed to a fall of pressure distal to the stenosis below that at the vertebralbasilar junction so that the pressure gradient in the vertebral artery is reversed. To our knowledge there has been no previous demonstration that vertebral-artery blood flow in man can be reversed as a result of a pathologic process.

> Willis[70] in his *Cerebri Anatome* (1664) postulated that in the carotid system the blood may enter via one side and on the other "haste backward by the same way, and to run back with an ebbing tide." It has, of course, been recognized by anatomists that the vertebral artery could serve as a collateral artery for the subclavian,[71] and to do this, the direction of flow in the vertebral artery would have to be brachiad rather than cephalad.

> Ligation of the subclavian artery may be required for therapeutic reasons in the treatment of traumatic lesions, of cyanotic congenital heart disease,[72] of coarctation of the aorta[73] or of aortic aneurysms. In such cases it appears preferable, if possible, to ligate the subclavian artery distal to the origin of the vertebral. If the subclavian must be ligated proximal to the vertebral, the vertebral artery should also be ligated. Otherwise, a reversal of blood flow through the vertebral artery will occur, and cerebral circulation will be reduced more than if the vertebral had been ligated and there was no flow through that vessel.[69]

In the same issue of the journal as the article by Reivich et al. there appeared an editorial by Fisher entitled "A New Vascular Syndrome— 'The Subclavian Steal.' "[74]

It is of interest to note that as early as 1837 it was realized that retrograde flow could take place through collateral channels into the distal portion of the subclavian artery beyond a more proximal occlusion.[75] Smyth (1866) reported the successful operation of a case of right subclavian aneurysm.[76,77] He also ligated the innominate and carotid arteries at the time of surgery and was forced to re-operate and ligate the vertebral artery because of hemorrhage. He stated:

> The ligation of the principal communicating branch with the distal end of a ligated artery, to arrest secondary haemorrhage from it, is an entirely new operation (the present instance of ligation of the vertebral being no doubt the first), and it is one of some value to general surgery.[77]

Smyth, in 1864, was also first to suggest that the "peculiarly rapid occurrence of syncope after bleeding" (at the operated site) was most likely the result of a retrograde current in the vertebral artery by way of communication with its fellow of the opposite side.[77]

We believe that the report from the Joint Study of 168 proven cases of subclavian steal represents the largest study published so far.[54] More than 80% of those patients also had associated lesions of other extracranial vessels. No significant difference in survival was found between those patients having surgery to extracranial vessels and those patients not subjected to surgery. Patients with only subclavian artery disease did not have strokes during the follow-up period, whether they were treated medically, surgically, or not at all.

Microsurgery and Bypass Operations

In 1960, Crawford et al. wrote concerning endarterectomy:

> The major limiting factor in the application of these procedures to small arteries has been lumen constriction resulting from arterial repair.[78]

In addressing this problem, Jacobson and colleagues (1962) described instrumentation and technique for microsurgical reconstruction of small arteries.[79] Two cases were reported in each of which an obstruction was removed from the middle cerebral artery for early hemiplegia. They stated:

> The surgery of arteries below 8–10 mm in size has been unsatisfactory because of the failure of patency, both early and late. This is in marked contrast to the successful surgery of larger arteries. It appeared that one possible explanation is that a smaller margin of allowable error in placement of sutures exists in the case of small vessels. It has been felt that the fault has not been the inability of the hand to perform, but rather the inability of the eye to guide the hand. The dissecting microscope, so essential to the middle ear surgeon, has been adapted to this purpose.[79]

Their paper had been presented at a meeting of the Harvey Cushing Society in 1961. In discussion, Dr. J. Lawrence Pool said that ten years previously he had done a bypassing procedure with Dr. Robert Merrick, "using a plastic tube to connect the superficial temporal artery with the anterior cerebral artery after the latter had been occluded following aneurysmal surgery. The tube successfully conducted blood from the external carotid system to that of the internal carotid system for at least an hour as we could see, and then, of course, later thrombosed. This patient, incidentally, is still alive and perfectly well in spite of this procedure!"[79]

On October 30, 1967, Yaşargil (Figure 4.6) performed a superficial temporal-to-temporal cortical artery shunt on a patient who had had an occlusion of the left middle cerebral artery (without collaterals) three months before the operation.[80] Follow-up angiography was refused, but pulsation of the superficial temporal artery remained good. On November 7, 1967, Yaşargil performed a similar procedure, and, in this instance, follow-up angiography showed that the bypass was patent. This surgery has become commonly known as extracranial–intracranial (EC-IC) bypass.

Also in 1967, Yaşargil first attempted to interpose an autogenous saphenous artery graft between the common carotid and middle cerebral arteries in dogs. In three animals used, all grafts were thrombosed when studied four to eight weeks later.[81]

Microsurgical reconstruction entailed the development of special instruments and ultrafine suture materials and needles. In 1970, Yaşargil et al. described end-to-side anastomosis between the end of the superficial temporal artery and the side of the temporal division of the middle cerebral artery in 9 patients.[82] In 11 cases, a direct arteriotomy was carried out in one or more segments of the middle cerebral artery with either embolectomy or thrombectomy being performed. Sutures were especially developed, No. 10–0 monofilament nylon, and 25X magnification was used.

In 1971, Lougheed et al. described common carotid to intracranial internal carotid bypass venous graft in a 54-year-old woman. They wrote:

> Frequently in carotid artery disease, one is faced with a totally occluded internal carotid artery that cannot be reopened. However, many of these cases have sufficient collateral circulation from the opposite carotid artery to nourish the affected hemisphere. It is not uncommon, though, to meet the situation where the carotid artery on the contralateral side is stenosed and this stenotic artery must supply both hemispheres. In such a situation, endarterectomy on the stenosed side carries with it a considerable risk. We attempted to avoid this risk by repairing the occluded side with a venous bypass graft from the common carotid artery in the neck to the internal carotid just distal to the anterior clinoid process. . . . The alternative method of connecting the superficial temporal artery to the middle cerebral artery does not supply as much blood as the larger bypass directly into the internal carotid artery.[83]

Although Yaşargil's saphenous artery grafts in dogs (1967) had not been successful, Maroon and Donaghy (1973) described their microsuturing techniques and also a new type of microtourniquet.[84] They reported cerebral revascularization with autogenous saphenous grafts in 14 dogs.

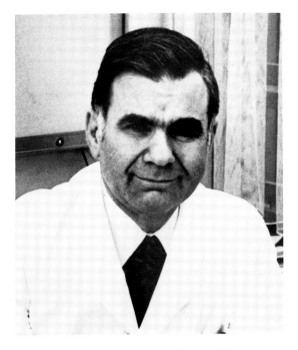

Figure 4.6. M. GAZI YAŞARGIL

Four of 6 saphenous artery grafts were patent when studied angiographically 4 to 70 days postoperatively; 3 of 8 venous grafts were patent when studied 1, 3, and 18 days following surgery. Maroon and Donaghy found obvious technical factors to account for all graft failures, stressed the importance of smooth approximation of the vessels, and emphasized that gentleness in handling and protection from drying are essential to success.

Also in 1973, Hunter and Donaghy described microautografts (arteries 1.0 mm or less in diameter) performed in rabbits using microsurgical techniques.[85] They stated:

> The neurosurgeon has attempted to improve cerebral blood flow in patients suffering from critical extracranial or intracranial occlusive vascular disease. Most common of these procedures has been the rotation arterial graft where a normal scalp vessel is dissected out, ligated and divided distally, and the distal end of the proximal segment is rotated into a new position and anastomosed to a cerebral vessel distal to the obstructing lesion. The superficial temporal artery-cortical artery anastomosis developed by Donaghy and Yaşargil is the best example of this procedure. Another method

uses a free, fresh venous autograft extending from the common carotid artery to the intracranial internal carotid artery, which bypasses the usual internal carotid artery occlusion in the neck (Lougheed et al.). Despite improved techniques, the occlusion rate of these and similar procedures remains high, and most failures occur in vessels of about 1 mm diameter.[85]

The authors described a series of 25 rotation and 25 free arterial grafts in rabbits, using vessels 1 mm or less in diameter, which were studied to delineate some of the factors that determined success or failure. The rotation grafts were successful in 21 of 25 (84%), while the free grafts were successful in 19 of 25 (76%). They used 25X magnification under the Zeiss binocular operating microscope. Most of the failures were due to infection or technical difficulties related to the construction of the suture line. They concluded that about 90% of arterial grafts of a diameter of 1 mm or slightly less will remain patent if the surgeon is trained and has an uncomplicated, noninfected situation.

EC-IC Bypass Study

By 1977, EC-IC bypass was in widespread use throughout the world, and an international cooperative study, supported by the U.S. National Institutes of Health, was initiated in order to test the value of the procedure. A randomized trial was designed to determine whether anastomosis of the superficial temporal artery to the middle cerebral artery could reduce subsequent stroke and stroke-related death among patients with symptomatic, surgically inaccessible (to endarterectomy) atherosclerotic stenosis or occlusion of the internal carotid or middle cerebral arteries.[86] To get the required number of patients, there were 71 centers on three continents. A total of 1377 patients participated; 714 randomly assigned to the best medical care, 663 assigned the same regimen with the addition of bypass surgery. Average follow-up was 56 months.

The outcome was surprising and unexpected by many because previously published reports on case series had documented improvement and positive results following bypass. However, the study showed that nonfatal and fatal stroke occurred both more frequently and earlier in the patients undergoing bypass surgery. Survival analyses comparing the two groups for major strokes and all deaths, for all strokes and all deaths, and for ipsilateral ischemic strokes demonstrated a similar lack of benefit from surgery. Also, TIAs occurred equally among medical and surgical patients.[87]

The trial design and methodology were highly commendable, and, remarkably, no patient was withdrawn or lost to follow-up. The postoperative patency rate was 96%, which certainly establishes the high degree of skill of the surgeons. Thirty-day surgical mortality and major stroke morbidity rates were 0.6% and 2.5%, respectively, figures comparable to those of experienced surgeons operating on similar patients at prominent medical centers. The results have a high level of statistical confidence, and there appears to be no reason to question them.

A possible explanation for the failure of bypass surgery to reduce mortality and morbidity is that the procedure itself could cause an increased risk of stroke or death. The bypass could actually facilitate the passage of emboli from proximal sites, and the disturbed flow dynamics in the middle cerebral artery bed might increase the risk of middle cerebral artery occlusion.[88]

References

1. Robicsek F: The medical history of extracranial cerebrovascular disease. In Extracranial Cerebrovascular Disease: Diagnosis and Management, Robicsek F (ed), New York, Macmillan, pp. 5–18, 1986.

2. Sloan HG: Successful end-to-end suture of the common carotid artery in man. Surg Gynec & Obstet 33:62–64, 1921.

3. von Parczewski S: Resection and anastomosis of the common carotid. Münch Med Wochenschr 63(46):1646, 1916.

4. von Haberer H: Wien klin Wchnschr xxxi(10):285, 1918.

5. Lexer: Muenchen med Wchnschr lxv:468, 1918.

6. Denk W: Wien klin Wchnschr xxxi:285, 1918.

7. Conley JJ, Pack GT: Surgical procedure for lessening the hazard of carotid bulb excision. Surgery 31:845–858, 1952.

8. Conley JJ: Free autogenous vein graft to the internal and common carotid arteries in the treatment of tumors of the neck. Ann Surg 137:205–214, 1953.

9. Foster JH: Arteriography—cornerstone of vascular surgery. Arch Surg 109:605–611, 1974.

10. Oudot J: La greffe vasculaire dans les thromboses du carrefour aortique. Presse Méd 59:234–236, 1951.

11. DuBost C, Allary M, Oeconomos N: Resection of an aneurysm of the abdominal aorta. Arch Surg 64:405–408, 1952.

12. Binswanger O, Schazel J: Beiträge zur normalen und pathologischen anatomie der arterieren des gehirns. Arch Psychiat 58:141, 1917.

13. Dow DR: The incidence of arteriosclerosis in the arteries of the body. Brit Med J 2:162–163, 1925.

14. Oppenheimer BS, Fishberg AM: Hypertensive encephalopathy. Arch Intern Med 41:264–278, 1928.

15. Spielmeyer W: Vasomotorisch trophische veränderungen bei zerebraler arteriosklerose. Mschr Psychiat 68:605, 1928.

16. Wolkoff K: Über atherosklerose der gehirnarterien. Bietr Z Path Anat Allg Path 91:515, 1933.

17. Keele CA: Pathological changes in the carotid sinus and their relation to hypertension. Quart J Med 2:213–220, 1933.

18. Sjøqvist O: Über intrakranielle aneurysmen der arteria carotis und deren beziehung zur ophthalmoplegischen migrane. Nervenarzt 9:233–241, 1936.

19. Johnson HC, Walker AE: The angiographic diagnosis of spontaneous thrombosis of the internal and common carotid arteries. J Neurosurg 8:631–659, 1951.

20. Moniz E, Lima A, de Lacerda R: Hémiplégies par thrombose de la carotide interne. Presse Méd. 45:977–980, 1937.

21. Leriche R, Fontaine R, Froehlich F: L'énervation sinu-carotidienne est-elle permise au point de vue physiologique? Presse Méd 43:1217, 1935.

22. Chao WH, Kwan ST, Lyman RS, et al: Thrombosis of the left internal carotid artery. Arch Surg 37:100–111, 1938.

23. Hultquist GT: Über Thrombose und Embolie der Arteria Carotis und hierbei vorkommende Gehirnstorungen. Jena, Gustav Fischer, 1942.

24. Fisher CM: Occlusion of the internal carotid artery. Arch Neurol Psychiat 65:346–377, 1951.

25. Fisher CM, Adams RD: Observations on brain embolism. J Neuropath & Exper Neurol 10:92–94, 1951.

26. Fisher CM: Occlusion of the carotid arteries: Further experiences. Arch Neurol Psychiat 72:187–204, 1954.

27. Ross RS, McKusick VA: Aortic arch syndromes: Diminished or absent pulses in arteries arising from the aortic arch. Arch Intern Med 92:701–740, 1953.

28. Carrea R, Molins M, Murphy G: Surgical treatment of spontaneous thrombosis of the internal carotid artery in the neck. Carotid–carotideal anastomosis. Acta Neurol Latinoamer 1:71–78, 1955.

29. dos Santos JC: Sur la désobstruction des thromboses artérielles anciennes. Mém Acad chir 73:409–411, 1947.

30. Leriche R, Kunlin J: Essais de désobstruction des artères thrombosées suivant la technique de Jean Cid dos Santos. Lyon chir 42:675–682, 1947.

31. Leriche R: Quatorze essais de thrombectomie artériel suivant la méthode de Jean Cid dos Santos; thrombo-endartériectomie désobstruante. Mém Acad chir 74:100–107, 1948.

32. Lemaire A, Reboul H, Loeper J: Endartériectomie désoblitérantes de l'aorte. Bull Soc méd hôp 65:656–660, 1949.

33. Bazy L, Huguier J, Reboul H, et al: Technique des "endartériectomies" pour artérites oblitérantes chroniques des membres inférieurs, des iliaques et de l'aorte abdominale inférieure. J chir 65:196–210, 1949.

34. Bazy L: L'endartériectomie pour artérite oblitérante des membres inférieurs. J internat chir 9:95–115, 1949.

35. Wylie EJ, Kerr E, Davies O: Experimental and clinical experiences with the use of fascia lata applied as a graft about major arteries after thrombo-endarterectomy and aneurysmorrhaphy. Surg Gynec & Obstet 93:257–272, 1951.

36. Wylie EJ: Thromboendarterectomy for arteriosclerotic thrombosis of major arteries. Surgery 32:275–292, 1952.

37. Strully KJ, Hurwitt ES, Blankenberg HW: Thromboendarterectomy for thrombosis of the internal carotid artery in the neck. J Neurosurg 10:474–482, 1953.

38. DeBakey ME: Successful carotid endarterectomy for cerebrovascular insufficiency: Nineteen year follow-up. JAMA 233:1083–1085, 1975.

39. Eastcott HHG, Pickering GW, Rob CG: Reconstruction of internal carotid artery in a patient with intermittent attacks of hemiplegia. Lancet 2:994–996, 1954.

40. Edwards C, Rob C: Relief of neurological symptoms and signs by reconstruction of a stenosed internal carotid artery. Brit Med J 2:1265–1267, 1956.

41. Cooley DA, Al-Naaman YD, Carton CA: Surgical treatment of arteriosclerotic occlusion of common carotid artery. J Neurosurg 13:500–506, 1956.

42. Fields WS, Crawford ES, DeBakey, ME: Surgical considerations in cerebral arterial insufficiency. Neurology 8:801–808, 1958.

43. Matas R, as cited in French LA, Haines GL: Unilateral vertebral artery ligation: Report of a case ending fatally with thrombosis of the basilar artery. Neurosurg 7:156–158, 1950.

44. Hutchinson EC, Yates PO: Cervical portion of vertebral artery: Clinicopathological study. Brain 79:319–331, 1956.

45. Hutchinson EC, Yates PO: Caroticovertebral stenosis. Lancet 1:2–8, 1957.

46. Crawford ES, DeBakey ME, Fields WS: Roentgenographic diagnosis and surgical treatment of basilar artery insufficiency. JAMA 168:509–514, 1958.

47. Cate WR, Jr., Scott HW: Cerebral ischemia of central origin: Relief by subclavian-vertebral artery thromboendarterectomy. Surgery 45:19–31, 1959.

48. Fields WS, North RR, Hass WK, et al: Joint study of extracranial arterial occlusion as a cause of stroke: Organization of study and survey of patient population. JAMA 203:955–960, 1968.

49. Hass WK, Fields WS, North RR, et al: Joint study of extracranial arterial occlusion: Arteriography, techniques, sites, and complications. JAMA 203:961–968, 1968.

50. Bauer RB, Meyer JS, Fields WS, et al: Joint study of extracranial arterial occlusion: Progress report of controlled study of long-term survival in patients with and without operation. JAMA 208:509–518, 1969.

51. Blaisdell WF, Clauss RH, Galbraith JG, et al: Joint study of extracranial arterial occlusion: A review of surgical considerations. JAMA 209:1889–1895, 1969.

52. Fields WS, Maslenikov V, Meyer JS, et al: Joint study of extracranial arterial occlusion: Progress report of prognosis following surgery or nonsurgical treatment for transient cerebral ischemic attacks and cervical carotid artery lesions. JAMA 211:1993–2003, 1970.

53. Heyman A, Fields WS, Keating RD: Joint study of extracranial arterial occlusion: Racial differences in hospitalized patients with ischemic stroke. JAMA 222:285–289, 1972.

54. Fields WS, Lemak NA: Joint study of extracranial arterial occlusion: Subclavian steal—a review of 168 cases. JAMA 222:1139–1143, 1972.

55. Gomensoro JB, Maslenikov V, Azambuja N, et al: Joint study of extracranial arterial occlusion: Clinical-radiographic correlation of carotid bifurcation lesions in 177 patients with transient cerebral ischemic attacks. JAMA 224:985–991, 1973.

56. Fields WS, Lemak NA: Joint study of extracranial arterial occlusion: Transient ischemic attacks in the carotid territory. JAMA 235:2608–2610, 1976.

57. Fields WS, Lemak NA: Joint study of extracranial arterial occlusion: Internal carotid artery occlusion. JAMA 235:2734–2738, 1976.

58. Blaisdell WF: Extracranial arterial surgery in the treatment of stroke. Proceedings of Eighth Princeton Conference. In Cerebral Vascular Diseases, McDowell FH, Brennan RW (eds), New York, Grune & Stratton, pp. 3–32, 1972.

59. Bruetman ME, Fields WS, Crawford ES, et al: Cerebral hemorrhage in carotid artery surgery. Arch Neurol 9:458–467, 1963.

60. Wylie EJ, Hein MF, Adams JE: Intracranial hemorrhage following surgical revascularization for treatment of acute strokes. J Neurosurg 21:212–215, 1964.

61. Warlow C: Carotid endarterectomy: Does it work? Stroke 15:1068–1076, 1984.

62. Shaw DA, Venables GS, Cartlidge NEF, et al: Carotid endarterectomy in patients with transient cerebral ischaemia. J Neurol Sciences 64:45–53, 1984.

63. Dyken ML, Pokras R: The performance of endarterectomy for disease of the extracranial arteries of the head. Stroke 15:948–950, 1984.

64. Dyken ML: Carotid endarterectomy studies: A glimmering of science. Stroke 17:355–358, 1986.

65. Whisnant JP: Role of neurologists in the decline of stroke. Ann Neurol 14:1–7, 1983.

66. Contorni L: Il circolo collaterale vertebrao-vertebrale nella obliterazione dell'arterio subclavia all sua origine. Minerva Chir 15:268–271, 1960.

67. Toole JF: Discussion. Proceedings of Third Princeton Conference. In Cerebral Vascular Diseases, Millikan CH, Siekert RG, Whisnant JP (eds), New York, Grune & Stratton, pp. 31–32, 1961.

68. Rob CG: Technique of surgical therapy. Proceedings of Third Princeton Conference. In Cerebral Vascular Diseases, Millikan CH, Siekert RG, Whisnant JP (eds), New York, Grune & Stratton, pp. 110–112, 1961.

69. Reivich M, Holling HE, Roberts B, et al: Reversal of blood flow through the vertebral artery and its effect on cerebral circulation. N Engl J Med 265:878–885, 1961.

70. Willis T: Cerebri Anatome: Cui Accessit Nervorum Descriptio et Usus. Londini, J Flesher, 1664.

71. Gray H: Anatomy: Descriptive and Applied. 22nd edition. London, Longmans, Green & Co. p. 636, 1923.

72. Blalock A, Taussig HB: Surgical treatment of malformations of heart in which there is pulmonary stenosis or pulmonary atresia. JAMA 128:189–202, 1945.

73. Shumacker HB: Use of subclavian artery in surgical treatment of coarctation of aorta. Surg Gynec & Obstet 93:491–495, 1951.

74. Fisher CM: A new vascular syndrome—"the subclavian steal." N Engl J Med 265:912, 1961.

75. Liston RL: Aneurism of the right subclavian artery (ligature of the subclavian and carotid arteries). Lancet 2:668–699, 1838.

76. Smyth AW: Successful operation in a case of subclavian aneurism. Original Communications, Art II, New Orleans Med Record, p. 4 (May 15), 1866.

77. Fields WS: Reflections on "The Subclavian Steal." Stroke 1:320–324, 1970.

78. Crawford ES, Beall AC, Ellis PR, et al: A technique permitting operation upon small arteries. Surg Forum 10:671–675, 1960.

79. Jacobson JH, II, Wallman LJ, Schumacher GA, et al: Microsurgery as an aid to middle cerebral artery endarterectomy. J Neurosurg 19:108–115, 1962.

80. Yaşargil MG: Microsurgery Applied to Neurosurgery. Yaşargil MG (ed), Stuttgart, Georg Thieme Verlag, pp. 108–109, 1969.

81. Yaşargil MG: Experimental small vessel surgery in the dog including patching and grafting of cerebral vessels and for formation of functional extra-intra-cranial shunts. In Microvascular Surgery, Donaghy RMP, Yaşargil MG (eds), Stuttgart, Georg Thieme Verlag, pp. 87–126, 1967.

82. Yaşargil MG, Krayenbuhl HA, Jacobson JH, II: Microneurosurgical arterial reconstruction. Surgery 67:221–233, 1970.

83. Lougheed WM, Marshall BM, Hunter M, et al: Common carotid to intracranial internal carotid bypass venous graft. J Neurosurg 34:114–118, 1971.

84. Maroon JC, Donaghy RMP: Experimental cerebral revascularization with autogenous grafts. J Neurosurg 38:172–179, 1973.

85. Hunter KM, Donaghy RMP: Arterial microautografts: An experimental study. Can J Surg 16:23–27, 1973.

86. EC/IC Bypass Study Group: The international cooperative study of extracranial/intracranial arterial anastomosis (EC/IC bypass) study: Methodology and entry characteristics. Stroke 16:397–406, 1985.

87. EC/IC Bypass Study Group: Failure of extracranial–intracranial arterial bypass to reduce the risk of ischemic stroke. N Engl J Med 313:1191–1200, 1985.

88. Editorial: Extracranial to intracranial bypass and the prevention of stroke. Lancet 2:1401–1402, 1985.

5

Medical Management
of Cerebrovascular Disease

In addition to the control of hypertension, diabetes, and cardiac abnormalities, specific anticoagulant or antiplatelet therapy has been tried in patients at risk for stroke.

Anticoagulant Therapy

Historical events in the development of anticoagulant therapy are interesting. Venesection was common in very early times, but the period of its inception is unknown. The use of leeches for healing was recorded in a medical encyclopedia written between 500 B.C. and A.D. 200. This Sanskrit document from India contained a full chapter on leeches.[1] The medical use of these parasites became popular in Europe, and in the 1700s a "leech express" transported them from Bavaria and Bohemia to France, where they were widely used until the present century. It is still not unusual in Europe to find leeches applied over the enlarged liver of a patient suffering from congestive heart failure. The pharmacists keep them in glass jars filled with water plus a little sand at the bottom. Here they remain unfed for months. In the 1960s it was reported that 4 million were used annually in Russia.[2]

Haycraft (1884) noted that bleeding from leech bites was difficult to stop.[3] At the beginning of this century the active anticoagulant ingredient in leech heads was isolated and Jacoby (1904) suggested the name "hirudin."[4] Sporadic work with hirudin was reported in 1929 and again in 1957, when it was isolated in crystalline form. Vigran (1965) stated, "The mechanisms of the prevention of thrombosis by Hirudin have not been studied, but now appear to be of historical interest only."[2]

However, as reported by Kennedy, with the recent advent of microsurgery in the reattachment of severed body parts, physicians are using leeches to help restore circulation.[1] For example, when a finger is reattached, the goal is to reestablish blood flow from and back to the heart. The outward flow is through arteries, which are relatively easy to suture. The arduous part of the operation is rejoining the smaller veins, which return blood to the heart. These veins are, of course, especially tiny in children. When the surgeon is unable to fully restore the venous drainage, blood becomes congested in the area of the wound, lowering the odds of a successful operation. When leeches are placed on the site, they draw out the congested blood while an anticoagulant in the leech saliva prevents clotting. After leeches are used for several days, the small severed veins naturally reattach themselves, greatly enhancing the likelihood of circulation adequate to maintain the part. The process is not painful because the saliva acts as a local anesthetic. Dr. Fred Valauri, a microsurgeon in San Francisco, said, "The leeches are like a godsend. They do everything a microsurgeon would want. If you wanted to design something, this is it. It's already been made. This is a fantastic ace in the hole." The market in the United States is large enough to support at least one business, Leeches USA, which supplies physicians and hospitals around the country. The blood-suckers are imported from Wales, where researchers are working to isolate the anticoagulant chemical from leech saliva and reproduce it in the laboratory for marketing as a pharmaceutical.[1]

In 1915, Jay McLean (Figure 5.1), a student at Johns Hopkins School of Medicine was given the task of isolating cephalin from brain tissue and determining if it had thromboplastic activity. It was believed that cephalin was possibly the thromboplastic substance in the body, but it could not be crystallized, and one could not be sure of its purity and hence its function. McLean reasoned that if the thromboplastic action in brain extract were due to some other substance, adherent to or absorbed by cephalin, this might not be so in organs that did not contain such a large amount of cephalin. He wrote:

In my reading of the German chemical literature on phosphatides, I found articles by Erlandsen and Baskoff in which they described extracts of heart and liver secured by a process similar to that for obtaining cephalin from the brain. Therefore, these products might be heart and liver cephalin, but were named cuorin (from the heart) and heparphosphatide (from the liver): hence the name "heparin."[5]

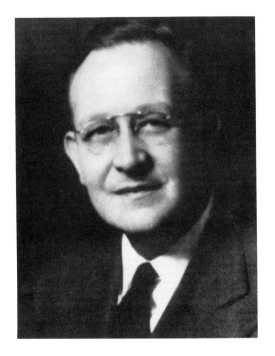

Figure 5.1. JAY MCLEAN
(From Vigran IM: *Clinical Anticoagulant Therapy*, 1965. Courtesy of Lea &
Febiger, Publisher, Philadelphia, PA)

McLean prepared these extracts:

> The various batches were tested down to the point of no thromboplastic
> activity, but two of those first prepared appeared not only to have lost their
> thromboplastic action, but actually to retard slightly the coagulation of the
> serum-plasma mixture. . . . I retested again and again until I was satisfied
> that an extract of liver (more than heart) possessed a strong anticoagulant
> action.[5]

A cat was bled and a batch of heparphosphatide added to the blood. The
blood never did clot.[5] A report of his work on isolating cephalin was
published in 1916.[6]

In 1918, Howell and Holt extended McLean's research.[7] They introduced, for the first time, the word "heparin" and found that it could also
be prepared from lymph glands.

In the 1920s, cattle in North Dakota and Alberta sometimes died from idiopathic internal hemorrhage or from blood seepage after minor injury or surgery. It was eventually deduced that the cause was the ingestion of improperly cured hay made from sweet clover and that the bleeding could be stopped by transfusing blood from normal cows. The clover feed resulted in a lowered level of a precoagulant substance, then labeled "prothrombin." The odor of the new-mown hay was due to a bitter compound named coumarin.[8,9] Link (Figure 5.2) and colleagues found that the natural coumarin in hay was transformed during spoilage to 4-hydroxycoumarin, two molecules of which were then coupled together to give a biscoumarin, which they named dicoumarol.[8] This was crystallized in 1939 and, over the next few years, Link's laboratory as well as pharmaceutical companies all over the world synthesized many related agents in order to identify those that could be used therapeutically.[9]

Around the same time, a Scandinavian, Per Hedenius (1941) wrote:

Figure 5.2. KARL PAUL LINK
(From Vigran IM: *Clinical Anticoagulant Therapy,* 1965. Courtesy of Lea & Febiger, Publisher, Philadelphia, PA)

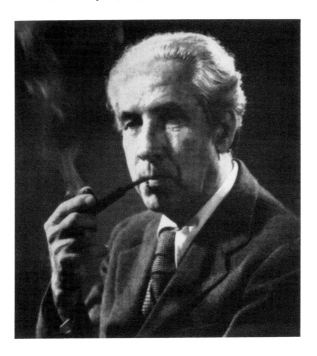

It will soon be 6 years since the—to my knowledge—first intravenous heparin injection was attempted on man. I made an injection on myself. In 1937–1938, I tried storage administration of heparin on experimental animals but found that in addition to other drawbacks it was necessary to double and redouble the size of the heparin dose in order to obtain an effect on the coagulation time. After Wilander and I had made our first experiments on the anti-coagulating effect of heparin on man, and had established that it was possible to fix the dosage with such precision that an expected effect could be obtained, the field was clear for clinical work.[10]

Hedenius and colleagues collected 85 cases treated with heparin, although 11 did not receive the dosage recommended by him. There were 10 cases of arterial embolism (6 to cerebral arteries), 33 cases of arterial thrombosis (20 cerebral or cerebellar), 38 cases of venous thombosis, and 4 cases of uncertain diagnosis. There was a favorable effect in 19 cases, no effect in 36, and uncertain effect in 30. He believed it was "obvious that this physiological anti-coagulant will in the future be useful as a reliable therapeutic medium in the treatment of thrombo-embolic disease."[10]

Rose was another early investigator in the use of anticoagulants for stroke.[11] In 1950, he related:

In most sites in the body thrombosis and embolic infarction are regarded as sufficient reasons for the use of anticoagulant drugs in their management. Infarction of the brain is a notable exception, and no account of the use of such measures in this condition has appeared in any of the more readily accessible journals. . . . [After a stroke] some recovery is the rule and this must mean that some of the immediate loss of function is the result of a temporary disturbance of fluid relationships around the area of infarction, and it has been postulated that there may be a spreading thrombotic process.[11]

He organized a clinical trial to test anticoagulant therapy in cases of acute stroke.

His design divided patients into three groups, and he recorded outcomes for each cohort. Group A comprised patients examined within 24 hours after the first symptoms of a stroke. They were given heparin and later, dicoumarol. In 10 of the 12 cases admitted in this category, the anticoagulants appeared to have no effect whatsoever. One patient recovered consciousness while on therapy but had such severe permanent disabilities from the stroke that the physician believed he had done the person a disfavor. A second patient died of cerebral hemorrhage on the ninth day when the prothrombin was around 30%. Group B included patients examined 24 to 48 hours after onset. They were given only dicoumarol. Of 6 cases in this classification, 2 had striking improvement, and no difference was noted in the other 4. There were no cerebral hemorrhages. Group C was composed of patients examined after 48 hours but within one week. They were also given only dicoumarol. None of the 6 patients appeared to have benefited. One patient died on the tenth day of a massive cerebral hemorrhage.

On the basis of these 24 cases, Rose concluded, "Use [of anticoagulants] is of no real value whatever."[11] He also made note of the fact that during the first 24 hours it is often difficult to make certain that a case is one of cerebral infarction and not hemorrhage.

Wright (1946) stated that 20 to 37% of episodes of myocardial infarction are destined to be followed by embolic or thrombotic complications.[12] Because the use of dicoumarol for the treatment of thromboembolic phenomena of the venous system had been attended by a striking reduction in the extension of thrombophlebitis, in the number of emboli encountered, and in the number of fatalities from emboli, he studied patients following myocardial infarction. He first used dicoumarol in 46 patients who were considered complicated cases. They had had multiple coronary thrombi within a period of one month, propagation of an original thrombus, or multiple emboli. They were classified as having a very serious prognosis, but 41 of 46 patients ceased having episodes as soon as they were under the effect of dicoumarol. Eleven died (24%). This figure was less than the estimated mortality of more than 60%. Eight died of cardiac failure as a result of their pretreatment massive infarctions. Wright then undertook treatment of 34 uncomplicated cases. These persons had had coronary thrombosis with infarction but otherwise had an uneventful course. On dicoumarol therapy, four died (12%). No mention was made of bleeding complications. In eight autopsies there was no evidence of hemorrhage.

Cosgriff (1950) described experiences of 17 patients (mainly with rheumatic heart disease and mitral stenosis), all of whom had had one or more emboli from an intracardiac source.[13] Dicoumarol was the principal therapeutic agent with heparin used only in the immediate period of one to four days after the acute embolus. During therapy, one patient suffered a pulmonary embolus and one a renal embolus. This latter person also had an embolus to the leg two and one-half months after stopping dicoumarol. Also, one patient had a fatal cerebral infarction 12 days after discontinuing dicoumarol, and a fourth patient had a pulmonary embolus one month after stopping the drug. The author concluded that continuous administration of an anticoagulant drug was feasible and safe.

Askey and Cherry (1950) prescribed anticoagulant therapy for 20 patients with heart disease and auricular fibrillation.[14] Treatment averaged 13 months. Eleven had excellent results, 7 fair results, and 2 were considered treatment failures. Complications ranged from pulmonary emboli (in one case) to hematuria and hematomas. The authors believed that "the incidence of thromboembolism appears to have been decreased."[14]

Around 1953, articles describing the use of anticoagulants for TIAs began appearing in journals. Campbell reported a case of vertebrobasilar insufficiency treated with Danilone® (phenylindandione, PID).[15] The patient had had five ischemic episodes, but these ceased and he had none during the eight-month period on therapy. Fisher and Cameron (1953) described a patient with incipient basilar artery thrombosis.[16] Repeated temporary attacks had occurred accompanied by an advancement of the neurologic deficit. Danilone was administered and for 33 days not a single attack was recorded. On cessation of therapy, episodes recurred and were banished again by either Danilone or heparin. The authors were puzzled:

> It is difficult to picture exactly a process which could lead to transient cerebral attacks and yet be prevented by anticoagulant therapy. The fact that heparin was as effective as PID indicates that hindrance of coagulation or thrombosis was an important factor in prevention of the attacks. . . .
>
> Transient phenomena preceding the onset of a stroke are much more frequent than is commonly believed, for the patient often neglects them, while his physician does not inquire about their occurrence once paralysis has occurred. In the field of cerebrovascular disease transient episodes nearly always reflect a thrombotic process, for intracerebral hemorrhage and cerebral embolism almost never occasion prodromal symptoms.[16]

Wright and McDevitt (1954) described anticoagulant therapy for the prevention of thromboemboli from a cardiac source.[17] In a long-term clinical trial with 57 patients, they found that during a period of 795 patient-months before anticoagulant therapy, there were 205 thromboembolic episodes, 81 of which were cerebral. After anticoagulation, during a period of 1162 patient-months, these same patients had 23 thromboembolic episodes, 6 cerebral.

Millikan et al. (1958) described 317 patients treated with anticoagulant drugs (heparin, ethyl biscoumacetate, bishydroxycoumarin).[18] The participants were divided into four categories: intermittent vertebrobasilar insufficiency, intermittent carotid insufficiency, vertebrobasilar thrombosis with infarction, and actively advancing occlusion of the carotid system. Of 179 treated patients with transient insufficiency, 172 had cessation of attacks; 9 deaths occurred in 107 treated patients with vertebrobasilar thrombosis with infarction; of 31 treated patients with advancing carotid symptoms, 29 had no further progression of neurologic deficits. The article made no mention of serious side effects.

Also in 1958, McDevitt et al. related the long-term effects of anticoagulant therapy in 100 patients with cerebral thrombosis or embolism.[19] There were hemorrhagic complications in 30 of these persons; 3 fatal cerebral hemorrhages. The authors concluded that anticoagulant therapy is effective in reducing the danger of recurrent thromboembolic episodes if contraindications are observed and prothrombin times are painstakingly controlled.

By the 1960s, heparin and dicoumarol were being used enthusiastically for cerebrovascular disease and a few small randomized trials were organized. Marshall and Shaw (1959) reported long-term PID therapy with 114 patients who had diffuse hemispheric disease, focal hemisphere "thrombosis," brainstem "thrombosis," or internal carotid artery occlusion.[20] There were 57 treated cases and 57 controls. At the end of 15 months, there were 3 deaths in the treated group (2 cerebral hemorrhages, 1 cardiac) and none in the control group. There were 5 further strokes (including the 2 fatal ones) in the treatment group and 2 in the control group.

In 1961, the Veterans Administration reported a randomized trial with 155 patients admitted from nine hospitals.[21] Patients with manifestations of either cerebral ischemia or cerebral infarction were divided equally between treatment and control therapy. These groups were observed on an average of 9 and 12 months, respectively. Of 78 treated patients, hemorrhagic complications occurred in 31 and resulted in 4 deaths; of 77 control patients, there were 5 bleeding complications with 1 death. Total mortality was 13 (16.7%) in the treated group; 7 (9.1%) in the control group. The authors concluded:

> Although anticoagulation appeared to decrease the number of attacks of ischemia, there was no reduction in the incidence of new or recurrent strokes. A higher mortality rate in treated patients was due in part to hemorrhagic complications.[21]

A trial among patients admitted to the neurology service at Bellevue Hospital (Groch et al., 1961) was composed primarily of cases of completed stroke.[22] In a randomized study, 92 persons were treated with dicoumarol or warfarin; 97 received no anticoagulant drugs. Controls were followed for 1615 patient-months; treated patients followed for 1996 patient-months (of which 892 patient-months were periods of satisfactory anticoagulant therapy). There were 20 bleeding episodes in the treated group (3 fatal), one episode in the control group (fatal cerebral hemorrhage). All hemorrhages were severe enough to warrant discontinuance of the anticoagulant. Deaths numbered 26 in the treated group, 35 in control. Fourteen of the control group deaths were caused by recurrent thromboemboli, while there were no deaths from this cause in the treated group during the period of anticoagulant therapy.

Pearce et al. (1965) randomly allocated 17 patients having TIAs to phenindione for 11 months and followed 20 control cases for 10.6 months.[23] Forty-one percent of treated patients and 55% of control patients had no further TIAs. This difference was not statistically significant. One person in each group sustained a nonfatal stroke and one control patient had a fatal stroke; 2 control patients died of cardiac causes. There were no major bleeding complications. The authors stated, "Though not absolutely conclusive, our results cast doubt on the value of anticoagulant treatment in transient cerebral ischaemic attacks."[23]

In 1966, Baker et al. reported a trial which included seven institutions and extended over 40 months.[24] Dicoumarol and heparin or dicoumarol alone were used depending on the length of time since the last ischemic episode. The patients had TIAs, thrombosis in evolution, thrombosis/ completed stroke, cerebral embolism, or "thorem" (a contraction of *th*rombosis or *em*bolism). The cases totaled 443; 219 in a control group, 224 in a treated group. The final opinion of the authors regarding survival:

> Judging from our data, it can be concluded that, from the standpoint of mortality, anticoagulant therapy plays no beneficial role in the treatment of thrombotic cerebrovascular disease and may be harmful.[24]

In the treated group, there were 12 fatal hemorrhagic complications, and hemorrhage contributed to a fatal outcome in a few further cases. Two instances of nonfatal intracerebral bleeding occurred in the treated group, one in the control.

Bradshaw and Brennan (1975) studied 49 patients who had sustained small strokes in the carotid territory and randomly allocated 25 of them to receive only supportive therapy and 24 to receive anticoagulant treatment.[25] Treatment times averaged 18 months. There was a reduced incidence of neurologic episodes during anticoagulant therapy, but after it was stopped, there was no significant difference between the two groups.

Although not a randomized trial, Whisnant et al. (1978) followed 199 patients having TIAs from the time of the first attack.[26] Those treated with anticoagulation showed no significant difference in survival from untreated patients.

None of the above articles called attention to the possibility that anti-coagulants might increase the risk of bleeding into atheromatous plaques leading to acute thrombosis. However, according to Sadoshima et al. (1979), this is a common postmortem finding. They stated:

> The frequent association of intramural hemorrhage and recent occlusive thrombosis indicates that both of these processes were in some manner causally related, or may be parallel effects or a combination of effects. The major cause of intramural hemorrhage was most likely bleeding from in-tramural small blood vessels which were connected with the arterial lu-mina. . . . These small blood vessels could develop in the course of or-ganization of the mural thrombus or progression of atherosclerosis.[27]

Also in 1979, Imparato et al. studied 69 carotid plaques removed at endarterectomy.[28] Stenoses were due to simple fibrous thickening in only 20%; the remainder were due to intraplaque hemorrhage, atheromatous debris, and, least often, luminal thrombus with or without ulceration. The authors concluded that carotid plaques start as fibrointimal thickening evolving to symptomatic stages by the occurrence of one or more of a number of pathologic changes, intraplaque hemorrhage being prominent.

Lusby et al. (1982) presented results of their study before the International Cardiovascular Society in Boston.[29] Investigation of carotid endarterectomy specimens showed that hemorrhage in atheromatous plaques plays a unique and major role in the development of cerebrovascular disease. Not only was intraplaque hemorrhage identified in most patients (92.5%) who exhibited symptoms, but a significant relationship was also established between the onset of symptoms and the development of plaque hemorrhage. During the discussion period, Imparato related that he and his colleagues had by this time analyzed 376 plaques; one-third had had microscopic hemorrhage within fibrous intimal thickening, one-third had had gross bleeding, and hemorrhage was the one factor that correlated most closely with the development of stenosis and probably ulceration.

The recognition that outcomes of trials using anticoagulants varied widely and that the randomized studies were small and had many faults in design and methodology was disconcerting to all physicians. Although anticoagulant therapy for cerebrovascular disease was popular for 15 to 20 years, particularly in a few large centers that had facilities for close supervision of prothrombin times, most physicians were relieved to see the advent of antiplatelet treatment which seemed much less hazardous.

Furthermore, in 1979, Furlan et al. reported that the general decline in the incidence of cerebral hemorrhage between 1945 and 1976 in Roch-

ester, Minnesota, was interrupted from 1961 to 1968 by "a dispropor-
tionately large number of intracerebral hemorrhages in patients treated
with anticoagulants."[30] Whisnant et al. had reported earlier that for patients 55 to 74 years old the risk of intracranial hemorrhage was increased
eight times in those treated by anticoagulation for TIA as compared with
untreated patients with TIA, and that all but one of their patients who
had intracranial hemorrhage had received anticoagulation for more than
one year.[26]

A final evaluation on the value of anticoagulant drugs for cerebrovascular disease has not, and cannot, be made. According to Warlow (1982),
an intelligent conclusion cannot be reached on the basis of published information. The randomized trials, even if combined, are not adequate in
quality or quantity for analysis. Cerebrovascular disease studies require
large numbers of patients for a long time or very large numbers for a
shorter time.[31]

The anticoagulant studies cited were accomplished in the era before
computed tomography (CT). Intracerebral hemorrhage can be diagnosed
much more accurately by CT than by the previous method of relying on
lumbar puncture. Small, circumscribed hemorrhages that did not communicate with the ventricles or subarachnoid space were often unrecognized. Kinkel and Jacobs (1976) found that cerebral infarction was the
clinical diagnosis in 43% of patients whose subsequent CT scans showed
hemorrhage.[32] Moreover, angiography was normal in 6 of 21 patients
with intracerebral hemorrhage. Therefore, some of the patients (in the
various anticoagulant trials previously described) who suffered intracerebral hemorrhage while receiving anticoagulant drugs may have been mis-
diagnosed originally and had bleeding before taking the drugs. The anticoagulant, of course, would tend to exacerbate the problem.

Heparin and the oral anticoagulant drugs inhibit fibrin formation and
although likely to interfere with venous thrombogenesis are rather less
likely to interfere with arterial thrombogenesis since platelets and not fibrin are the primary component of arterial thrombi.[31] Anticoagulants are
used in patients with a cardiac source of embolism, but the ratio of risk
to benefit is not known.[33]

The whole question of the value of anticoagulants has been reactivated
recently by the publication of results of a randomized, double-blind study
in Holland (898 postmyocardial infarction patients), which showed that
anticoagulation significantly reduced total deaths and deaths attributed to
recurrent myocardial infarction. Also, an excess of hemorrhagic strokes
in the treated group was more than balanced by a reduction in nonhem-

orrhagic strokes.[9,34] Therefore, in spite of the fact that the focus during the last decade has been on antiplatelet therapy, we may not have seen the end of the anticoagulant controversy.

Antiplatelet Therapy

Although many compounds alter platelet aggregation, aspirin has been the logical choice for long-term therapy in humans because it is a relatively safe, inexpensive substance with a long history of use by a high percentage of the population, and because its effect lasts for the life of the exposed platelet. To our knowledge, Lawrence L. Craven (1950) (Figure 5.3) was the first to report the use of aspirin for prophylaxis of thrombosis.[35] He knew that dental patients sometimes experienced hemorrhage after tooth extraction because aspirin in the blood stream precluded formation of the necessary clot. Craven urged male friends and patients to take one or two aspirin tablets daily. In 1950, he reported his results with aspirin prophylaxis in 400 men; in 1953, he published a summary of administration to 1465 males;[36] and, in 1956, he described the prevention

Figure 5.3. LAWRENCE L. CRAVEN
(Courtesy of Glendale News Press, Glendale, CA)

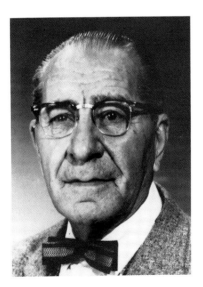

of coronary and cerebral thrombosis in 8000 men with use of 5 to 10 grains of aspirin daily.[37] Craven stated, "Not a single case of detectable coronary or cerebral thrombosis has occurred among patients who faithfully have adhered to this regime."[37] In the introduction to his 1956 publication, he wrote:

> Increasing emphasis on the atherosclerotic component in cardiovascular disease apparently has blinded many physicians to the fact that thrombosis, the process whereby the lumen of a vessel is occluded by a clot, is due primarily to an increase in coagulation rate of the blood. True, factors such as the narrowing of a vessel's lumen by the atherosclerotic process, or the action of large-sized cholesterol molecules in the circulation may have a contributing influence; nevertheless, in the last analysis the thrombotic episode is based upon formation of the clot.
>
> For many years physicians successfully have prevented or at least reduced the number of thrombo-embolic episodes in their patients by administering heparin, coumarin derivatives, or phenyl-indanedion drugs, whose sole effect is to depress or slow the coagulation rate. We physicians have, in effect, waited until after the initial damage has been done and then attempted to prevent further damage. In this paper I should like to suggest a simple but surprisingly effective means of altering the coagulation rate so as not only to forestall secondary attacks but also to prevent the initial thrombotic attack.[37]

He also had experimented with administration of a small dose of dicoumarol (10 mg daily) to 45 persons who were intolerant of or hypersensitive to salicylates. He believed that this limited experience suggested that a small amount of dicoumarol may also afford effective prophylaxis.

This report by Craven appeared in an obscure medical journal and was not widely disseminated. It was 20 years before interest in aspirin for thrombosis was revived. By 1970, research of blood platelets had clarified their function in thrombogenesis. Two reports of limited experience with aspirin for TIAs appeared in 1971:

1. Harrison and colleagues related that aspirin, 600 mg daily, had stopped frequent attacks of amaurosis fugax in two patients.[38]
2. Mundall et al. reported the disappearance of episodes of transient monocular blindness in a patient who was treated with aspirin, 600 mg four times daily.[39] This patient also had thrombocytosis, and her platelets aggregated spontaneously in vitro. On aspirin therapy, aggregation returned to normal.

By this time, physicians were more cognizant of the value of the randomized clinical trial in determining the worth of a drug or treatment modality, and, in the early 1970s, the first aspirin studies were organized.

AITIA Study

The Aspirin in Transient Ischemic Attacks Study was a randomized double-blind trial composed of two groups of patients: (1) those who had had attacks of monocular blindness (amaurosis fugax), hemisphere TIAs, or minor strokes (medical group); and (2) those with similar histories who had carotid endarterectomy before entering the trial (surgical group). Patients were randomly allocated to either aspirin (650 mg twice daily) or placebo and followed to determine the incidence of subsequent TIAs, death, cerebral infarction, or retinal infarction. Nonfatal myocardial infarctions were also recorded but these numbers were not cited in the publications.[40,41]

In the total group (303 patients from 10 participating centers), there was no statistically significant differential between the aspirin and placebo treatments when endpoints were restricted to death or cerebral or retinal infarction. In the medical group of 178 patients, there was a significant difference in favor of aspirin when subsequent TIAs were included as endpoints. This significance was most apparent in two subgroups of patients—those with a history of multiple TIAs and those with carotid lesions appropriate to their TIA symptoms. In the surgical cohort of 125 patients, life table analysis that eliminated deaths that were not stroke-related revealed a significant difference in favor of aspirin.

CCSG Trial

The Canadian Cooperative Study Group enlisted 585 patients from 12 centers in Canada. Individuals were randomly allocated to one of four regimens: sulfinpyrazone 200 mg 4 times daily, aspirin 325 mg 4 times daily, both drugs, or placebo. Among patients treated with aspirin alone, there were 22 strokes during follow-up versus 20 in the placebo group. However, for the total patient population, aspirin reduced the risk of stroke or death by 31% (48% among males). Among women, there were more hard endpoints (strokes and deaths) for the aspirin takers than for those not receiving the drug (17 vs. 12).[42]

AICLA Study

In 1975, Accidents Ischemiques Cerebraux Liés à l'Atherosclerose was undertaken to determine whether aspirin (1 g/day) or aspirin plus dipyridamole (225 mg/day) would produce a significant reduction in the occurrence of fatal and nonfatal cerebral infarction after 3 years of follow-up. On the basis of the results (cerebral infarcts totaled 31 in the placebo group, 17 in the aspirin group, 18 in the aspirin plus dipyridamole group), the authors concluded that aspirin had a significantly beneficial effect that was not enhanced by dipyridamole. They found no difference between males and females in the response to aspirin.[43]

Danish Trial

Patients (203) who had experienced at least one reversible cerebral ischemic attack of less than 72 hours duration were randomly assigned to treatment with either aspirin 1000 mg daily (101 patients) or placebo (102 patients). Patients referred for carotid surgery were excluded from the trial; this course may have eliminated many individuals who would be expected to benefit from aspirin, i.e., those with appropriate ulcerated lesions. The average follow-up was 25 months, and the results were reported in 1983.[44] No statistically significant differences were found between the treatment groups for stroke or death. The occurrence of TIAs was not reduced by aspirin. Angiography was performed on only 37 of the patients on aspirin and 25 of the placebo patients. There was relevant carotid stenosis in only 13 patients on aspirin and 3 placebo patients. Thus, the proportion of patients with normal carotid arteries was higher than that in other studies. Also, 24 aspirin and 31 placebo patients discontinued the trial without having reached an endpoint, leaving only 77 aspirin and 71 placebo patients. As emphasized previously, these numbers are too small to test the effectiveness of a drug for patients with cerebrovascular disease.

UK-TIA Aspirin Study

Between 1979 and 1985, 2435 patients with a history of TIA, amaurosis fugax, or minor stroke were randomly allocated to one of three regimens: aspirin 300 mg daily, aspirin 600 mg twice daily, or placebo. Endpoints included stroke, first myocardial infarction, or vascular death. A total of 1621 patients received aspirin, and 814 were allocated to the control group. There were 348/1621 endpoints among the treated patients, and 204/814 among those receiving a placebo (21.5% vs. 25%). Nonfatal strokes were 139/1621 and 92/814 (8.6% vs. 11.3%). There was no significant difference between the therapeutic benefits of low-dose and high-dose aspirin.[45]

The final answer to the question regarding the optimal dose of aspirin in vascular disease is awaited. Several controlled trials are under way. One, in particular, in the Netherlands is testing a very low dose against the doses used in previously reported studies of patients with TIAs and minor strokes.

References

1. Kennedy JM: Blood-sucking leeches discovering new niche as a microsurgery aid. Los Angeles Times as reported in the Houston Chronicle, June 29, 1987.

2. Vigran IM: Clinical Anticoagulant Therapy. Philadelphia, Lea & Febiger, 1965.

3. Haycraft JB: On the action of a secretion obtained from the medical leech on the coagulation of blood. Proc Roy Soc London 36:478, 1884.

4. Jacoby C: Über Hirudin. Deutsche med Wchnschr 30:1786, 1904.

5. McLean J: The discovery of heparin. Circulation 19:75–78, 1959.

6. McLean J: The thromboplastic action of cephalin. Am J Physiol 41:250–257, 1916.

7. Howell WH, Holt E: Two new factors in blood coagulation—heparin and pro-antithrombin. Am J Physiol 47:328–341, 1918.

8. Link KP: The discovery of dicumarol and its sequels. Circulation 19:97–107, 1959.

9. Mitchell JRA: Anticoagulants in coronary heart disease—retrospect and prospect. Lancet 1:257–262, 1981.

10. Hedenius P: Use of heparin in internal disease. Acta Med Scand 107:170–177, 1941.

11. Rose WM: Anticoagulant in management of cerebral infarction: Record of poor result obtained. M J Australia 1:503–504, 1950.

12. Wright IS: Experiences with dicoumarol in the treatment of coronary thrombosis with myocardial infarction. Tr A Am Physicians 59:47–50, 1946.

13. Cosgriff SW: Prophylaxis of recurrent embolism of intracardiac origin: Protracted anticoagulant therapy on ambulatory basis. JAMA 143:870–872, 1950.

14. Askey JM, Cherry CB: Thromboembolism associated with auricular fibrillation: Continuous anticoagulant therapy. JAMA 144:97–100, 1950.

15. Campbell MH: Basilar artery syndrome. Canad M A J 69:314–315, 1953.

16. Fisher CM, Cameron DG: Concerning cerebral vasospasm. Neurology 3:468–473, 1953.

17. Wright IS, McDevitt E: Cerebral vascular disease: Significance, diagnosis, and present treatment, including selective use of anticoagulant substances. Ann Int Med 41:682–698, 1954.

18. Millikan CH, Siekert RG, Whisnant JP: Anticoagulant therapy in cerebral vascular disease—current status. JAMA 166:587–592, 1958.

19. McDevitt E, Carter SA, Gatje BW, et al: Use of anticoagulant in treatment of cerebral vascular disease. JAMA 166:592–596, 1958.

20. Marshall J, Shaw DA: Anticoagulant therapy in cerebrovascular disease. Proc Roy Soc Med 52:547–549, 1959.

21. Veterans Administration: An evaluation of anticoagulant therapy in the treatment of cerebrovascular disease. Neurology 11 (2):132–138, 1961.

22. Groch SN, McDevitt E, Wright IS: A long-term study of cerebral vascular disease. Ann Int Med 55:358–367, 1961.

23. Pearce JMS, Gubbay SS, Walton JN: Long-term anti-coagulant therapy in transient cerebral ischaemic attacks. Lancet 1:6–9, 1965.

24. Baker RN, Broward JA, Fang HC, et al: Anticoagulant therapy of cerebral infarction: Report of a national cooperative study. In Cerebrovascular Disease, Proceedings of Association for Research in Nervous and Mental Disease, Millikan CH (ed), Baltimore, Williams and Wilkins, pp. 287–302, 1966.

25. Bradshaw P, Brennan S: Trial of long-term anticoagulant therapy in the treatment of small stroke associated with a normal carotid angiogram. J Neurol Neurosurg Psychiat 38:642–647, 1975.

26. Whisnant JP, Cartlidge NEF, Elveback LR: Carotid and vertebral-basilar transient ischemic attacks: Effect of anticoagulants, hypertension, and cardiac disorders on survival and stroke occurrence—a population study. Ann Neurol 3:107–115, 1978.

27. Sadoshima S, Fukushima T, Tanaka K: Cerebral artery thrombosis and intramural hemorrhage. Stroke 10:411–414, 1979.

28. Imparato AM, Riles TS, Gorstein F: The carotid bifurcation plaque: Pathologic findings associated with cerebral ischemia. Stroke 10:238–245, 1979.

29. Lusby RJ, Ferrell LD, Ehrenfeld WK, et al: Carotid plaque hemorrhage. Arch Surgery 117:1479–1488, 1982.

30. Furlan AJ, Whisnant JP, Elveback LR: The decreasing incidence of primary intracerebral hemorrhage: A population study. Ann Neurol 5:367–373, 1979.

31. Warlow C: Transient ischaemic attacks. In Recent Advances in Clinical Neurology, Matthews WB, Glaser GH (eds), Edinburgh, Churchill Livingstone, pp. 191–214, 1982.

32. Kinkel WR, Jacobs L: Computerized axial transverse tomography in cerebrovascular disease. Neurology 26:924–930, 1976.

33. Easton JD, Sherman DG: Management of cerebral embolism of cardiac origin. Stroke 11:433–442, 1980.

34. Sixty Plus Reinfarction Group: A double-blind trial to assess long-term oral anticoagulant therapy in elderly patients after myocardial infarction. Lancet 2:989–994, 1980.

35. Craven LL: Acetylsalicylic acid, possible preventive of coronary thrombosis. Ann Western Med & Surg 4:95–99, 1950.

36. Craven LL: Experiences with aspirin (acetylsalicylic acid) in the nonspecific prophylaxis of coronary thrombosis. Mississippi Valley M J 75:38–44, 1953.

37. Craven LL: Prevention of coronary and cerebral thrombosis. Mississippi Valley M J 78:213–215, 1956.

38. Harrison MJG, Marshall J, Meadows JC, et al: Effect of aspirin in amaurosis fugax. Lancet 2:743–744, 1971.

39. Mundall J, Quintero P, von Kaulla K, et al: Transient monocular blindness and increased platelet aggregability treated with aspirin—a case report. Neurology 21:402, 1971.

40. Fields WS, Lemak NA, Frankowski RF, et al: Controlled trial of aspirin in cerebral ischemia. Stroke 8:301–316, 1977.

41. Fields WS, Lemak NA, Frankowski RF, et al: Controlled trial of aspirin in cerebral ischemia. Part II: Surgical group. Stroke 9:309–319, 1978.

42. Canadian Cooperative Study Group: A randomized trial of aspirin and sulfinpyrazone in threatened stroke. N Engl J Med 299:53–59, 1978.

43. Bousser MG, Eschwege E, Haguenau M, et al: "AICLA" Controlled trial of aspirin and dipyridamole in the secondary prevention of atherothrombotic cerebral ischemia. Stroke 14:5–14, 1983.

44. Sørensen PS, Pedersen H, Marquardsen J, et al: Acetylsalicylic acid in the prevention of stroke in patients with reversible cerebral ischemic attacks. A Danish Study. Stroke 14:15–22, 1983.

45. Antiplatelet Trialists' Collaboration: Secondary prevention of vascular disease by prolonged antiplatelet treatment. Br Med J 296:320–331, 1988.

6

Noninvasive Vascular Studies

Many noninvasive techniques for examining the carotid artery bifurcation have been developed over the past 30 years. These methods have been used singly or in diverse combinations to delineate the extent and characteristics of atherosclerotic disease. However, the clinical significance of diagnosed abnormalities and the necessity for therapeutic intervention remain debatable topics. Approximately 30 to 40% of autopsies show some degree of carotid stenosis that, often, is an incidental finding. Carotid stenosis may be a harbinger of stroke for one patient, whereas an apparently identical lesion in another patient may never cause symptoms.[1]

All of these noninvasive methods have been judged by comparison with arteriography, and only a few recently developed techniques, such as magnetic resonance imaging (MRI), radionuclide imaging with indium-111 labeled platelets, and scanning with late-model duplex equipment, appear to have the capacity to allow consistent diagnosis of small ulcerated plaques. Noninvasive tests, however, may be even more effective than arteriography in monitoring hemodynamic changes distal to the cervical carotid bifurcation.[2]

Cerebral Blood Flow Measurement

In 1885, Fick assessed cardiac output by measuring arteriovenous differences of carbon dioxide and oxygen along with oxygen uptake or carbon dioxide production.[3] In 1924, Haggard postulated that the rate at which an anesthetic gas is taken up by the brain depends in part on the rate of blood flow in that organ.[4] In 1945, Kety (Figure 6.1) and Schmidt used both of these concepts to plan a series of experiments to measure

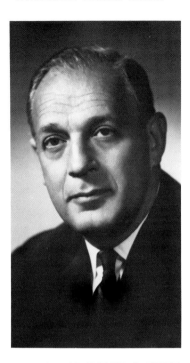

Figure 6.1. SEYMOUR S. KETY
(Courtesy of National Institutes of Health Archives Collection, 1962. Edward A. Hubbard, photographer)

blood flow to the brain.[5] The Fick principle expressed the idea that the quantity of a substance taken up by the brain equals the total amount of the substance brought to it by the arterial blood minus the quantity taken away by the venous blood for the same period.[3,6] Kety and Schmidt stated that quantitative measurements of the total blood flow to the brain of man had not been reported previously. Their method was based on the assumption that the rate at which the cerebral venous blood content of an inert gas approaches the arterial blood content depends on the volume of blood flowing through the brain.[5]

They had subjects breathe 15% nitrous oxide while samples from an artery and from the jugular bulb were simultaneously drawn. They measured the nitrous oxide uptake of the brain and calculated cerebral blood flow. Their method measured the average perfusion rate of the brain in ml per 100 g of perfused brain tissue per minute.[7] Lassen (1964) said,

"The fundamental limitation of the inert gas inhalation method lies in the fact that uneven perfusion of the brain tissue causes a certain underrepresentation of slowly perfused tissue areas with the result that the flow value is somewhat overestimated."[7]

In 1955, Lassen and Munck (Denmark) published a new method for determining cerebral blood flow with radioactive krypton according to the Kety and Schmidt principle.[8] In 1956, Greitz (as cited by Nylin) had a different approach: the radiologic study of brain circulation by rapid serial angiography, two pictures per second, measuring the circulation time, i.e., the time difference between the points of maximum concentration in the carotid siphon and the parietal veins.[9] He also made controls injecting radioactive iodine-131. Greitz achieved the same results with the two methods for measuring circulation time. In 1964, Lassen wrote:

> Diffusible radioactive indicators, such as the gases krypton-85 or xenon-133, cross the blood-brain barrier freely. There are ample theoretical and experimental reasons to believe that such indicators reach essentially diffusion equilibrium in one single transit of the capillary blood through the corresponding tissue cylinder. This means that the uptake and elimination of such indicators is actually rate-limited only by the blood flow. With the radioactive gas dissolved in normal saline, the tracer can be directed to the brain by intra-arterial injection. This approach has two advantages: First, by injecting into the internal carotid or vertebral artery, the tracer reaches the brain practically exclusively. Second, at the end of the injection, the isotope concentration in the arterial blood drops almost instantaneously to zero. The examination is carried out most conveniently in conjunction with cerebral angiography, since access to the cerebral arterial tree is then already assured. The injection of the saline containing the radioactive gas does not give rise to subjective or objective symptoms, and the radiation exposure is a small fraction of exposure involved in one single conventional X-ray photograph of the skull.
>
> The concentration of isotope in various regions of the injected part of the brain is followed by external scintillation detectors. . . . A preliminary study of 7 subjects studied with the injection of krypton-85 into the vertebral artery indicated a blood flow in the human cerebellar area of about half that in the hemispheres.[7]

Other substances that have been used subsequently to measure either total or regional cerebral blood flow include hydrogen, antipyrine labeled with iodine-131, and water labeled with oxygen-15. Most methods require puncture or catheterization of either the jugular bulb or internal carotid artery, with attendant discomfort and risk to the patient.[10] Xenon-133 was also administered through inhalation by Conn (1955)[11] and by

Mallett and Veall (1963).[12] This avoids catheterization, but the indicator is delivered to extracerebral structures as well as to the brain and recirculates in the blood. Consequently, the clearance curves obtained from the head must be subjected to elaborate analysis with a computer to separate the brain contribution from that of the scalp and skull.[10]

Both cerebral blood flow and metabolism have recently been studied by a variety of methods that involve tomographic measurements. Xenon in conjunction with computed tomography (CT) provides highly detailed cerebral blood flow measurements. As anatomic resolution improves with CT and MRI, an understanding of the physiologic changes accompanying or preceding morphologic changes is necessary for their correct interpretation.[13] Detailed mapping of brain blood flow has so far been restricted to invasive experiments in animals. Investigators have used radionuclide-labeled microemboli[14,15] of diffusible substances such as iodoantipyrine that equilibrate in tissue.[16-19] With these methods valuable information has been obtained about normal cerebral blood flow and the changes brought about by such conditions as ischemia, edema, hemorrhage, tumors, and degenerative disease. Researchers have also been able to discern the responses of collateral circulation to ischemia and the pattern of infarction to be expected after a specific stroke.[13] By using these advanced techniques, it becomes apparent that motor activation of a hand immediately increases flow within the appropriate region of the motor strip on the opposite side, and that visual stimulation activates the occipital region,[20,21] whereas deprivation of a specific sensory input is associated with significant reductions of flow in appropriate regions.[13] When noninvasive methods of local flow measurement in humans become widely available, the study of brain function in both normal and diseased states will be significantly stimulated.

Ophthalmodynamometry

The ophthalmodynamometer was introduced in 1917 by Bailliart and others and was utilized chiefly by European ophthalmologists to study ocular cirulation in different eye diseases.[22,23] Antin and Karlan state, "While it was also used for studying retinal vascular dynamics, there was no suggestion of its role in interpreting and diagnosing lesions produced by cerebrovascular disease."[23] It was the German ophthalmologist Baurmann who, in 1936, first described the phenomenon of lowered pressure in the retinal artery of the side of an occluded carotid artery.[23,24] It was not until the early 1950s that ophthalmodynamometry received attention in the

American literature as a simple, safe, and reliable technique in the diagnosis of carotid artery disease.[23]

In 1953, Thomas and Petrohelos reported on the diagnostic significance of retinal artery pressure in internal carotid artery lesions.[25] In 1956, Svien and Hollenhorst described the use of Bailliart's instrument and the method they used in studying patients.[26] They found that over 90% of persons without neurologic or ocular disease had essentially equal retinal artery pressures in both eyes. However, after occlusion of the internal carotid artery, a significant difference in pressure resulted and was maintained indefinitely. After ligation of the common carotid artery, a significant difference resulted, but did not persist. Presumably, in the latter case, collateral flow from the external carotid to the internal carotid was augmented over time and resulted in nearly normal blood pressure in the internal carotid artery.

In 1961, at the Third Princeton Conference on Cerebrovascular Diseases, Hollenhorst stated:

> The problem with ophthalmodynamometry is that in about 30% of patients with carotid occlusive disease, readings are equal on the two sides. Retinal pressures do not aid in diagnosis. In about 6% of our series, the retinal artery pressure is elevated on the side of the involved carotid instead of lowered.[27]

Fluorescein Arm to Retina Time

At the same Princeton Conference, Heyman (1961) reported a new ophthalmoscopic procedure for the diagnosis of cerebrovascular disease.[28] He injected fluorescein dye into an arm vein and measured the time until its appearance in the retinal arterial circulation. In patients with carotid artery obstruction, there is a delay in the appearance time of the dye in the ipsilateral retinal arterioles as seen by ophthalmoscopic examination. With bilateral carotid occlusion, the test has less value. This technique had been described previously by Novotny and Alvis (1960),[29] but had not been specifically applied to occlusive cerebrovascular disease.

Oculosphygmography

In 1964, Bynke and Krakau described a "handy instrument for oculosphygmography"[30] and two years later Bynke wrote:

Several investigators[31-33] have pointed out that the amplitude of pulse-synchronous variations of the intraocular pressure is reduced on the side of carotid occlusion. . . . The intraocular pressure varies synchronously with the pulse. It is probable that the main cause of these variations is the pulsatile blood flow of the choroid, which is known to contain the principal portion of the intraocular blood volume.

The pressure variations are transmitted via the cornea and the plunger of the instrument to the piezoelectrical crystal. This leads to flexions and deflexions of the crystal, the other end of which is fixed. In this way, variations in electrical potential are produced, which are then conducted directly to the recorder.

Diagnostic value is equivalent to ophthalmodynamometry. However, as oculosphygmography is objective and more rapid, does not require much training, and has a greater applicability, it has proved superior.[34]

Thermography

Simple bolometers have been used for many years by astronomers to measure heat from stars. The thermograph was developed in connection with space exploration and is a motor-driven scanning thermalresistor bolometer that also detects heat spontaneously emitted by various objects. Wood explains that "a thermogram is a two-dimensional photographic image obtained by two to four minutes of scanning and comprises approximately 60,000 individual heat recordings. The thermograph operates at a distance from the patient and detects and records only radiant heat spontaneously emitted from the body surface."[35]

One method of assessing blood flow in any portion of the body is by determining the temperature of that part and recognizing a variation from the physiologic state. In the case of the limited external display of the internal carotid artery, sensitive instruments are required to demonstrate a variation of skin temperature from the normal.[35]

In 1965, Wood reported his experience with thermography, testing 1000 subjects to establish normal values and then applying the technique to 117 patients with intra- or extracranial cerebrovascular abnormalities. A significant difference in temperature was not evoked with lesions of the internal carotid artery until that vessel was 50 to 60% closed. Then, blood flow through the ophthalmic artery was usually reduced, resulting in skin cooling. The medial supraorbital skin exhibits changes more consistently than the globe of the eye or the medial canthus. These latter areas are also supplied by branches of the external carotid and, therefore, tend to remain warm. The medial supraorbital area of the forehead is the only portion of the facial skin supplied by terminal branches originating from the internal carotid artery.[36] Wood found an abnormal forehead pattern in 88% of patients with occlusive or stenotic lesions of that vessel.[35]

Ocular Plethysmography

In 1963, Lawrence et al. developed a technique for utilizing the ophthalmic pulse as a monitor of blood flow in the ophthalmic artery during common or external carotid compression and were able to demonstrate collateral pathways in 11 patients with known internal carotid occlusions.[37,38] The safety and simplicity of this method suggested to Brockenbrough et al. (1967) a wider application in the evaluation and management of patients with suspected carotid obstruction.[38]

They monitored phasic changes in the volume of the eye (produced by pulsatile blood flow) by means of a plastic cup attached by gentle suction to the sclera and connected through a fluid-filled system to pressure transducers. The main source of blood supply to each eye could be identified by briefly compressing each neck vessel in turn and observing the response of the ophthalmic pulses. Since the method is based on changes in ocular volume, it was termed "ocular plethysmography" and the authors initially tried it with 77 patients.

Subsequently, other investigators described clinical application of the saline-filled system,[39,40] but Gee et al. (1974)[41] believed that it had limitations and could be improved. They had an instrument manufacturer construct a bilateral ocular pneumoplethysmograph (OPG) which incorporated transducers and a pneumatic system specifically designed for its intended use. The equipment was compact, portable, air-filled instead of saline-filled, and designed for bilateral simultaneous application and for simultaneous recording of intracerebral blood pressure.

Hays et al. (1972) had previously reported on the use of carotid "stump" pressure as an indicator of the adequacy of collateral circulation to the ipsilateral cerebral hemisphere during carotid clamping for endarterectomy.[42] This experience suggested to Gee and colleagues that similar information, if it could be obtained preoperatively by a noninvasive technique, would be of value in choosing patients for surgery. They stated:

> We used the ocular pneumoplethysmograph to obtain tracings during alternate compression of each common carotid artery to assess the adequacy

of collateral circulation to each eye (and its respective cerebral hemisphere). By this means we hope to predict the fate of that hemisphere if the internal carotid artery becomes occluded, either from progress of stenosis or during operative clamping for arterial repair.[41]

They presented findings in over 300 examinations.

Phonoangiography

Kartchner and McRae (1969) developed an audiovisual method for the investigation of the characteristics of carotid bruits to enhance clinical auscultation and screening of patients for arteriography.[43] A specially adapted microphone was applied over the cervical carotid arteries at low, middle, and high levels to make audiorecordings of carotid bruits. The recordings were analyzed for the degree of underlying stenosis. The highest level corresponded to the bruit emanating from the occlusive lesion. The middle recording further confirmed the presence of a significant bruit or might even reveal a barely audible bruit not detected at the highest position. The lowest recording confirmed the presence or absence of a bruit originating from a cardiac murmur or a stenotic lesion at the aortic arch level.

Kartchner et al. (1973) used two complementary techniques—carotid phonoangiography and oculoplethysmography—to evaluate 360 carotid arteries in 208 patients. When compared with arteriography, they determined that a composite diagnostic accuracy of 86% by phonoangiography and 91% by oculoplethysmography was achieved. A saline-filled instrument was used in the latter procedure.[44]

Ultrasonic Doppler Methods

The phenomenon of Doppler[45] refers to the frequency shift that arises when a wave source and a receiver are in movement relative to one another in the same or in the opposite direction of the wave propagation path.[46] An ultrasonic Doppler method for detecting blood flow without cannulating the vessels examined was first described by Franklin et al. in 1961. They reported:

> The Doppler shift of ultrasound, scattered from moving elements within a stream of blood, is related to the velocity of blood flow. A flowmeter based

on this principle has been constructed and was used to record blood flow through intact vessels of dogs.[47]

Ultrasonic directional flowmeters utilizing the Doppler principle were first used on the carotid vessels in 1965 by Miyazaki and Kato. They reported hemodynamic comparisons of right and left carotid arteries in patients with hemiplegia.[48]

Müller states:

> In 1966, Stegall et al.[49] described an ultrasonic flow detector based on the Doppler effect that permitted the recording of pulse curves indicating changes of blood flow velocity through intact human skin. With this technique the blood corpuscles are used as ultrasound reflectors. If the transducer is placed over a blood vessel at an angle other than orthogonal, the velocity of the blood corpuscles has a vector in the direction of the sound beam, and, thus, a pulsatile Doppler frequency shift is produced.[46]

The value for neurologic diagnosis is limited because the external and internal carotids cannot be examined separately as they may be superimposed. A similar difficulty arises when the vertebral artery is examined. Though fairly reproducible Doppler signals generally are obtained when the transducer is positioned over this vessel, one cannot be certain of registering a solely vertebral artery signal due to the superimposed occipital branches of the external carotid.[46]

A new approach to obtain information about the internal carotid circulation was tried by Maroon et al. (1969).[50] These investigators did Doppler recordings by placing the transducer on the closed eyelid and, using a nondirectional flow detector, recorded both intensity and Doppler shift frequency in time caused by the streaming in the ophthalmic artery. They demonstrated internal carotid occlusions quite clearly. However, they pointed out that false-normal or controversial findings may be obtained in patients having good collateral circulation from the external carotid via the facial and anterior temporal arteries, with reversed flow through the ophthalmic artery. This occurrence could possibly give the same trace as a physiologic circulation. Logically then, Maroon's technique was modified with a directional ultrasonic flow detector.[46] Müller (1972) described his method of directional Doppler sonography applied at the ophthalmic artery, which allowed the recognition of flow reversal in 14 of 15 cases of internal carotid thrombosis and in 6 of 12 cases of highgrade internal carotid stenosis.[46]

By 1972, a number of reports had been published concerning the application of ultrasonic directional flowmeters in the assessment of intra- and extracranial carotid blood flow; however, no carotid artery imaging was performed.[51] In 1972, Reid and Spencer linked the flow probes to a position-sensing arm and thus recorded an ultrasonic angiogram or image of the carotid artery and its bifurcation. They stated:

> The present ultrasonic Doppler flow detectors that use the Doppler effect on waves scattered from moving blood have provided useful information when directed by hand to trace the circulation of animals and man. By scanning with a highly directive flow detector, the areas of flow can be localized. Images can be formed of the interior of blood vessels. These images have the appearance of arteriograms and venograms made by dye contrast radiography, but have none of its hazards. The resolution appears adequate for useful images.[52]

Pulse Echo Ultrasound

In general, ultrasonic applications in vascular disorders are divided into two large groups: (1) Doppler ultrasound and (2) pulse echo (reflected) ultrasound. The first of these is designed primarily to provide information about flow within a vessel, and the second concerns producing an actual image of the vessel.[53]

In the simplest form of display, the echo reflections are shown as vertical deflections on the oscilloscope screen, with the strength of the echo indicated by the height of the deflection. This is termed "amplitude modulation" or A-mode.[53]

Kristensen et al. (1971) applied A-mode ultrasound scans to the internal carotid artery in 325 patients and gave an evaluation of the method on the basis of comparison with 166 angiograms of the artery. They stated:

> If the method were used for selection of patients for angiography, 5% of operable lesions would be missed while 30% with nonoperable conditions would be referred to angiography. When combined with other methods of investigation (ophthalmodynamometry, oculosphygmography, thermography, etc.), these percentages can be lowered.[54]

With B-mode ultrasound recording, the echo pulse is not shown as a spike, but is reduced to a dot on the oscilloscope screen. The strength of the echo is no longer indicated by its amplitude but rather by its brightness. This is termed "brightness modulation" or B-mode.[53]

Olinger (1969) (Figure 6.2), one of the participating investigators in the Joint Study of Extracranial Arterial Occlusion, recognized that the employment of "4-vessel angiography" to screen patients for vascular surgery carried with it both pain and risk and at that time required hos-

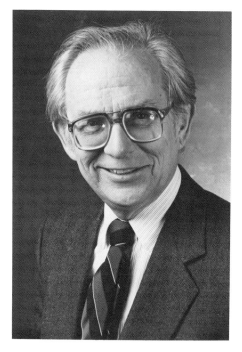

Figure 6.2. CHARLES P. OLINGER

pitalization.[55] Furthermore he pointed out that both expensive radiographic equipment and skilled personnel were required. Moreover, arteriography failed to show an operable lesion in about 25% of the cases and was not suitable for repeat studies during long-term evaluation of the operative results or medical management. Olinger believed that "what is needed is a safe and simple pre-stroke screening system to visualize extracranial vascular disease."[55] Influenced by the earlier work of Hertz,[56] who used ultrasound to visualize the chambers of the heart, and Howry and Bliss,[57] who were the first to demonstrate a cross-sectional view of a carotid bifurcation, Olinger published one of the first reports on the visualization of the carotid arteries by B-mode ultrasound technique (Figure 6.3). He believed that the method had potential for detecting extracranial occlusive disease before a stroke and for long-term evaluation of atherosclerosis and its treatment.[55]

Blue et al. (1972) evaluated 30 carotid arteries by ultrasonic B-mode scanning, and the results were correlated with those of conventional arteriography.[58] The most reliable criterion for identification of the internal carotid artery was the serrated pattern produced by arterial pulsation. The absence of the pattern was a good indication of a significantly stenotic lesion. In their series, there was a 73% correlation between scans and arteriograms. Three scans were false positive. The fact that there were no

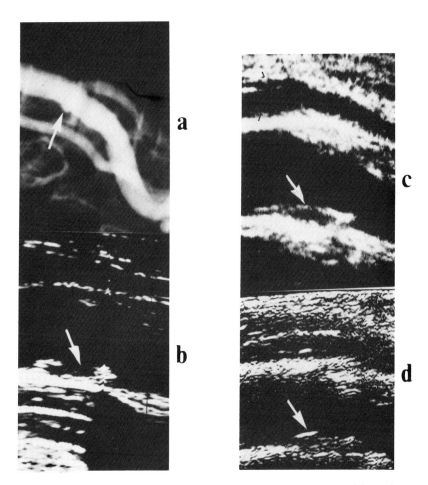

Figure 6.3. Patient, presented following TIA, was placed on aspirin and remained asymptomatic. Carotid arteriogram (a) at baseline, demonstrating ulcer (arrow). Ultrasonic images at (b) one month, (c) three months, (d) six months, as it slowly healed. (Previously unpublished photographs, with permission of Charles P. Olinger)

false negative scans indicated to the authors that B-mode scanning was a useful screening procedure in the evaluation of patients suspected of having extracranial vascular disease. With the B-scan system, some lesions cannot be imaged because they are "sonically translucent"; that is, they have the same acoustical impedance as the moving blood. A B-scan image of a vessel with such a lesion may demonstrate what appears to be a normal lumen.[59]

In 1971, Hokanson et al. used a pulsed Doppler velocity detector to produce an ultrasonic arteriograph.[60] Because of the ability to select the depth of flow recording, the pulsed Doppler arteriograph was more discriminating than the continuous-wave devices and was capable of providing both longitudinal and horizontal cross-sectional views.[61]

In 1976, Sumner et al., from the same group, reported that their original instrument had been modified by incorporating 6 range gates for more rapid scanning, a single 3 mm piezoelectric crystal for improved resolution, and a direction-sensing capability to eliminate confusion from venous flow.[62] They compared ultrasonic arteriograms and roentgenograms of 81 carotid arteries. All occluded arteries and all stenoses greater than 50% were correctly identified. False positive ultrasonic arteriographs were obtained in 11% of the studies (believed due to sound absorption of calcifications in the arterial wall). False negative arteriographs (from plaques and ulcerations less than 1 mm in size) occurred in 22% of the studies.

Lusby et al. (1981) published a prospective evaluation of pulsed Doppler imaging.[63] Seventy-six carotid bifurcations of 39 consecutive patients who were undergoing investigation of TIAs were studied prospectively, using both pulsed Doppler imaging and X-ray contrast angiography. Pulsed Doppler imaging detected 93% of lesions seen, including most of those of less than 50% stenosis. The lateral Doppler scan was an important addition in the detection of disease. However, ulceration distal to a tight stenosis went undetected by pulsed Doppler.

Russell (1984) stated, "The major limitations [of pulsed Doppler ultrasonic arteriography] are the subjective nature of the test and the need for an experienced examiner. Several months of experience are usually required before an individual can correctly assess normal and abnormal flow signals and produce accurate images."[64]

Transcranial Doppler Ultrasound

Although the described techniques of Doppler ultrasound have been used successfully in the diagnosis of extracranial arterial obstructive lesions, the application of noninvasive ultrasound for measurement of intracranial cerebral arterial flow has been unsatisfactory, mainly because bone mass reduces the penetration of ultrasound. The resultant weak reflections make adequate recordings of blood flow velocities from intracranial arteries impossible.[65]

In 1982, Aaslid et al. introduced a high-energy bidirectional pulsed Doppler system operating at lower frequencies, which enables reliable measurement of flow velocity from cerebral arteries at the base of the skull.[66] They believe the technique will be useful for evaluation of the cerebral circulation in vascular occlusive disease as well as for the detection of vasospasm after subarachnoid hemorrhage.[65,67,68]

Hennerici and colleagues (1987) scanned 50 presumed healthy persons in different age classes to establish normal reference values.[65] They identified the intracranial carotid, middle cerebral, anterior cerebral, posterior cerebral, intracranial vertebral, and basilar arteries. They suggested using measurements of mean flow velocities, as they (1) are less influenced by high flow velocity, but low amplitude, signals originating from small vessels near the main arteries under consideration, (2) react less to minor flow inhomogeneities on the vessel wall, and (3) are less affected by frequently occurring pulse rate differences. Hennerici et al. stated, "The advantages of transcranial Doppler examination are its noninvasive, easily reproducible approach for the detection of rapid alterations of blood supply within the major cerebral arteries, which is impossible with other techniques available today."[65]

Duplex Scanning

Blackshear et al. (1979) described the duplex scanner.[69] It produces a B-mode image combined with pulsed Doppler spectrum analysis. By using the ultrasonic image as a guide for precise placement of the pulsed Doppler sample volume, the characteristics of blood flow can be determined at points of interest in the carotid arteries.

On a B-mode scan, it often is impossible to distinguish a noncalcified plaque or thrombus from blood. In a trial of a high-resolution B-mode scanner at the Mayo Clinic, this inability to detect the fatty plaque or thrombotic occlusion contributed to diagnostic errors in over one-third of the examinations.[69,70]

Ultrasonic imaging alone can be misleading. Wall calcification, which inhibits the transmission of ultrasound, may prevent the detection of flow in an area where, in fact, the vessel is patent, thus leading to an erroneous diagnosis of an occlusion or stenosis. The sample volume, with the duplex system, can be placed precisely at any point across the arterial diameter. The B-mode component provides a real time image of the artery in any desired plane, from which the flow velocity patterns may be evaluated.[69]

Accuracy with the duplex scanner is particularly good in patients with bilateral high grade stenoses or occlusion. These lesions have been most difficult to identify with noninvasive methods that rely on the detection of pressure and flow discrepancies compared to the contralateral carotid system. Blackshear et al. reported, "In our studies, the correct diagnosis was made in every case."[69]

Fell et al. (1981) reported a series of 750 patients (with suspected extracranial carotid arterial disease) evaluated with their duplex scanner.[71] Cerebral arteriography was also done on 135 (18%) of these individuals. The degree of stenosis was measured independently and was available for comparison with the results of duplex scanning and spectral analysis. Duplex scanning correctly detected the presence of disease in 252 of 259 carotid artery studies (97%). The extent of involvement varied from plaques that produced less than 10% diameter reduction to those that resulted in total occlusion. The technique was less accurate with lesions that produced less than 10% diameter reduction.

Bluth et al. (1986) used a high-resolution duplex scanner to study the carotid arteries of 50 patients before these patients underwent endarterectomy.[72] The plaques were evaluated carefully by vascular surgeons and pathologists for intraplaque hemorrhage. Sonography was accurate in identifying the presence or absence of hemorrhage in 90% of the cases. The authors believe that this method may ultimately be useful in determining patients at risk for emboli. As discussed in Chapter 5, several vascular surgeons, including Imparato et al.[73,74] and Lusby et al.,[75] have found a significantly increased incidence of intraplaque hemorrhage in their symptomatic patients as compared with those who were asymptomatic. It is considered possible that intraplaque hemorrhage may be the precursor to embolic phenomena.[72]

In a review of the noninvasive diagnosis of extracranial cerebrovascular diseases, Lees and Kistler (1984) stated, "Used alone and in combination with other techniques, this instrument [the duplex Doppler] has been increasingly successful for the accurate diagnosis of carotid disease."[76] However, the vertebral arteries, because of their size and location, have not been particularly amenable to diagnosis with this instrument. The major drawbacks to the duplex scanner are its expense, complexity, and relatively costly upkeep. Also, only the neck region can be studied; intracranial disease is undetected. However, it appears to be the ultrasound method of choice in laboratories with sufficient test volume to warrant its use.

Computed Tomography (CT)

On April 19, 1972, at the Annual Congress of the British Institute of Radiology, Hounsfield of the Central Research Laboratories of EMI, Ltd. spoke:

> For many years past, X-ray techniques have been developed along the same lines, namely, the recording on photographic film of the shadow of the object to be viewed. Recently, it has been realized that this is not the most efficient method of utilizing all the information that can be obtained from the X-ray beam. Oldendorf (1961)[77] carried out experiments based on principles similar to those described here, but it was not then fully realized that very high efficiencies could be achieved and so, picture construction techniques were not fully developed.[78]

Hounsfield (Figure 6.4) originated the concept that the use of a computer could permit recovery of an abundant amount of information concerning soft tissues which had previously been lost, due to superimposition of data and insensitivity of traditional methods of recording radiographic images.[79]

The prototype equipment was tested on patients with a wide variety of pathological conditions at Atkinson-Morley's Hospital for approximately 18 months, and James Ambrose, neuroradiologist at that institution, also spoke at the same Annual Congress. He described the scanning of the cranium in successive layers by a narrow beam of X-rays, in such a way that the transmission of the X-ray photons across a particular layer could be measured, and by means of a computer, used to construct a picture of the internal structure. Ambrose stated:

> It is possible that this technique may open up a new chapter in X-ray diagnosis. Previously, various tissues could only be distinguished from one another if they differed appreciably in density. In this procedure, absolute values of the absorption coefficient of the tissues are obtained. The increased sensitivity of computerized X-ray section scanning thus enables tissues of similar density to be separated and a picture of the soft tissue structure within the cranium to be built up.[80]

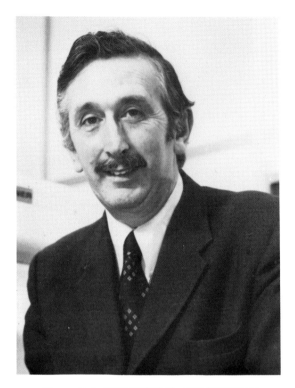

Figure 6.4. GODFREY N. HOUNSFIELD

The system outlined was considered to be approximately 100 times more sensitive than conventional X-ray, and a complete cranial study consisted of 28,000 absorption values which were analyzed by density.[79]

Knowledge of this new neuroradiologic capability soon spread worldwide, and in June 1973 the first EMI scanner in North America was installed at the Mayo Clinic; in July 1973 the second was in operation at Massachusetts General Hospital.[79] Between August 1973 and April 1974, more than 750 patients had CT at the latter institution. Brains from 10 of these subjects were sectioned. Nearly exact correlation was found between the anatomic location and extent of intracranial lesions demonstrated by CT and the findings on gross and microscopic examination.[81]

The major impact of CT scanning in assessment of cerebrovascular disease is its ability to detect intraparenchymal hemorrhage and intracranial lesions that may mimic stroke.[82] Sandercock et al. (1985) stated that CT provides useful information in a minority (up to 28%) of patients with first stroke and that scanning all persons with stroke would be prohibitively expensive.[83] Approximately 96,000 individuals in England and Wales have a first stroke every year. It is more practical to select only those whose management is likely to be influenced by investigation. The authors believe that the stroke patients who should have CT can be selected by the following simple criteria: (1) doubt (usually because of an inadequate history) as to whether the patient has had a stroke or has a treatable intracranial lesion; (2) the possibility of cerebellar hemorrhage or infarction; (3) the exclusion of intracranial hemorrhage in patients who either are already taking or likely to need antihemostatic drugs or are being considered for carotid endarterectomy; and (4) patient deterioration in a fashion atypical of stroke.

These guidelines seem to be appropriate for health care systems directed toward maximal cost efficiency. In the United States, physicians tend to recommend at least a noncontrast CT scan for every patient with a suspected central nervous system lesion (vascular or otherwise). It is not unusual to encounter patients in whom the first clinical impression is "cerebral thrombosis," but who are ultimately diagnosed as having intracerebral hemorrhage, subdural hematoma, tumor, etc. Also, the pattern of the infarct, i.e., lacunar or wedge-shaped, helps determine the pathophysiologic basis of the stroke and, therefore, helps guide workup and therapy. Contrast CT may be necessary to detect arteriovenous malformations and to exclude tumor, etc., in selected patients.

CT scanning suggests that in most patients with TIAs, study results will be normal and that in patients who have suffered stroke, scans will show abnormal findings in at least 48 hours.[84] Recently, CT has been used for direct assessment of the cervical carotid arteries to define carotid calcification in patients with TIAs.[85] In a small series, all 17 patients with TIAs and angiographically abnormal arteries showed carotid calcification on CT scans of the neck. Of three patients with normal arteries, the cervical tomograms showed normal findings.[85]

Magnetic Resonance Imaging (MRI)

Nuclear magnetic resonance, a physical phenomenon exhibited by certain atomic nuclei, was independently discovered by Bloch et al.[86] at Stanford University and Purcell et al.[87] at Massachusetts Institute of Technology in 1946. Bloch (Figure 6.5) and Purcell (Figure 6.6) shared the Nobel Prize in Physics in 1952. Nuclear magnetic resonance was originally used

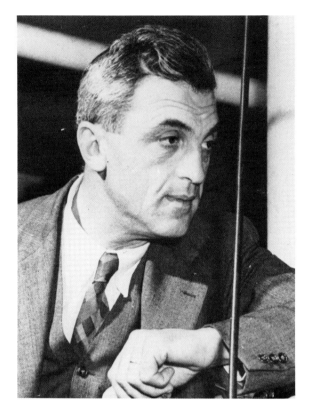

Figure 6.5. FELIX BLOCH
(From Wide World Photographers and Associated Press)

as a spectroscopic approach to determine chemical structure.[88] More recently, it has been applied to medical imaging, making possible high-resolution three-dimensional images based on the proton density of various structures (magnetic resonance imaging).

Infarcted brain tissue may be detected earlier by MRI than by CT, and the former may better quantitate the amount of edema and the extent of the infarction.[89] CT scanning can often discern the site of infarction in the thalamus, subthalamus, occipital lobe and/or cerebellum, but when infarction occurs in the brainstem, obscuration by bone artifact limits the usefulness of CT. However, MRI can reliably document infarcted tissue in the brainstem; in addition, by documentation of the extent and location of the infarct, the etiology may be suggested, i.e., whether large or small vessel disease is responsible.[90]

Ruszkowski et al. (1985) reported:

> The potential use of MR imaging for the clinical evaluation of the carotid arteries has recently been demonstrated. Because of the tortuous route of the carotid artery, previous attempts by others to image the area of the bifurcation in a single plane have been unsuccessful. The use of oblique plane imaging has enabled us to visualize the course of the carotid artery from the common carotid through the area of its bifurcation to the internal and external carotids. Dynamic blood flow within the vessels has been demonstrated throughout the course of the carotid. Clinical studies have shown that the anatomic as well as the physiologic status of the carotid can be evaluated using this method of MR imaging-carotid angiography.[91]

Disease of the arteries can now be detected with MRI and other techniques (positron emission tomography, radioisotope imaging) before end-organ damage, such as brain infarction or brain hemorrhage, occurs. Ar-

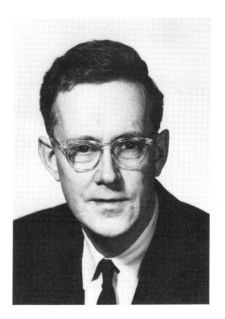

Figure 6.6. EDWARD MILLS PURCELL
(From Wide World Photographers and Associated Press)

terial atheroma can be imaged by MRI, and the expected improvements in the resolution of this technique, along with the development of appropriate contrast agents, may make MRI a very valuable aid in the diagnosis of preclinical carotid atherosclerosis so that preventive rather than symptomatic therapy can be applied.[76] In addition, the presence of fatty deposits and calcified areas in the arterial wall can be detected by MRI.[92]

High field MRI can also be used to determine cerebral venous thrombosis since the evolution and resolution of the entire venous occlusive process can be followed.[93]

Positron Emission Tomography (PET)

The first positron computed tomograph was developed by Phelps et al. (1975).[94−96] This system was referred to as the PETT II (positron emission transaxial tomograph).[97] Correia et al. (1985) state:

> An important strength of PET is that it measures physiologic disturbances, which in some disease states, such as epilepsy and psychiatric disorders, may occur in the absence of anatomic lesions; in others, such as acute stroke and Huntington's disease, it anticipates the development of such lesions; and in tumors, where a structural lesion is present, it may serve to metabolically characterize the lesion. An additional and very powerful use of PET involves the study of normal physiology, for example, the activation of various brain structures in response to sensorimotor or cognitive stimuli such as visual and auditory stimulation.[98]

A major hindrance to the widespread use of PET scanning is the expense; it requires a cyclotron. It has been estimated that equipment and space for a PET center costs between $3.5 and $5 million, while annual operating expenses are at least $1.2 million.[99]

Radionuclide Imaging

This has been used recently to detect the localization on arterial lesions of autologous platelets labeled with indium-111. Thakur et al. introduced the indium-111 oxine technique for labeling platelets in 1976,[100] and it has been tested over the cervical carotid bifurcation, comparing results with contrast arteriography. Indium-111-labeled platelets accumulate on atherosclerotic plaques to a degree sufficient for scintigraphic display of these lesions. Davis et al. (1978) reported that labeled platelets accumulated in vascular lesions (in some patients) despite anticoagulant or antiplatelet therapy.[101] They were able to detect bilateral ulcerated carotid plaques in one patient and venous thrombosis in two other patients. The authors believe that this technique shows promise as a noninvasive means of diagnosing focal atherosclerotic or thombotic lesions.

This is a much simpler and less expensive method than PET or MRI, and equipment for the performance of such nuclear medicine studies is available in virtually every hospital.[76] However, some authors believe that this technique is too insensitive for detection of any but the most obvious lesions.[92,102] Also only a low dose of indium-111 can be used due to its long half-life.[92] By contrast, studies show that low-density lipoprotein, the major cholesterol-carrying protein, concentrates strongly in healing experimental arterial lesions and can be used to image asymptomatic as well as symptomatic arteriosclerosis in humans.[76] Lees et al. used low-density lipoproteins labeled with indium-125 as tracers to identify atherosclerotic lesions in the carotid artery of the neck.[103] They based their investigations on the fact that metabolic changes in the arterial wall are common in the early phases of atherosclerosis, and these alterations are characterized by cellular proliferation and accumulation of low-density lipoprotein in the arterial wall. They examined three subjects with known disease confirmed by angiography and one control who had no focal low-density lipoprotein accumulation.

Lees and Kistler state:

> Further improvements in radiopharmaceuticals and in the instrumentation used for imaging should result in a simple and relatively inexpensive method for detecting early and/or metabolically active foci of arterio-sclerosis, which may be preferential sites of embolization or of acute arterial occlusion. These and other related methods may make noninvasive and nonarteriographic methods the preferred techniques for diagnosis of cerebrovascular disease within the next 10 to 20 years.[76]

References

1. Eastcott HHG: The results of surgical treatment of transient ischemic attacks: Lessons for future case selection. Int Surg 69:215–221, 1984.

2. Ackerman RH: Noninvasive diagnosis of carotid disease in the era of digital subtraction angiography. Neurol Clin 1:263–278, 1983.

3. Posner JB: Newer techniques of cerebral blood flow measurement. Proceedings of Eighth Princeton Conference. In Cerebral Vascular Diseases, McDowell FH, Brennan RW (eds), New York, Grune & Stratton, pp. 145–162, 1972.

4. Haggard HW: The absorption, distribution and elimination of ethyl ether. J Biol Chem 59:771–778, 1924.

5. Kety SS, Schmidt CF: The determination of cerebral blood flow in man by the use of nitrous oxide in low concentrations. Am J Physiol 143:53–66, 1945.

6. Fick A: Silzungsb. d. phys.-med. Gesellsch. zu Würtzb, p. 16, 1870.

7. Lassen NA: Various definitions of cerebral blood flow. Proceedings of Fourth Princeton Conference. In Cerebral Vascular Diseases, Millikan CH, Siekert RG, Whisnant JP (eds), New York, Grune & Stratton, pp. 56–61, 1964.

8. Lassen NA, Munck O: The cerebral blood flow in man determined by the use of radioactive krypton. Acta Physiol Scand 33:30–49, 1955.

9. Nylin G: Estimation of cerebral blood flow and cerebral blood pool by the aid of labelled erythrocytes. Proceedings of Second Princeton Conference. In Cerebral Vascular Diseases, Wright IS, Millikan CH (eds), New York, Grune & Stratton, pp. 40–52, 1958.

10. Report of the Joint Committee for Stroke Facilities. VI. Special procedures and equipment in the diagnosis and management of stroke. Stroke 4:111–137, 1973.

11. Conn HL, Jr.: Measurement of organ blood flow without blood sampling. J Clin Invest 34:916–917, 1955.

12. Mallett BL, Veall N: Investigation of cerebral blood flow in hypertension, using radioactive xenon inhalation annd extracranial recording. Lancet 1:1081–1082, 1963.

13. Wolfson SK, Jr., Yonas H, Gur D: Local cerebral blood flow imaging with stable xenon. In Noninvasive Diagnostic Techniques in Vascular Disease, Bernstein EF (ed), St. Louis, C.V. Mosby, pp. 269–288, 1985.

14. Dole WP, Jackson DL, Rosenblatt JI, et al: Relative error and variability in blood flow measurements with radiolabeled microspheres. Am J Physiol 243:H371–378, 1982.

15. Wagner HN, Rhodes BA, Sasaki Y, et al: Studies of the circulation with radioactive microspheres. Invest Radiol 4:374–386, 1969.

16. Eklöf B, Lassen NA, Nilsson L: Regional cerebral blood flow in the rat measured by the tissue sampling technique: A critical evaluation using four indicators C^{14}-antipyrine, C^{14}-ethanol, H^3-water and xenon^{133}. Acta Physiol Scand 91:1–10, 1974.

17. Kennedy C, Des Rosiers MH, Sakurada O, et al: Metabolic mapping of the primary visual system of the monkey by means of the autoradiographic (^{14}C) deoxyglucose technique. Proc Natl Acad Sci USA 73:4230–4234, 1976.

18. Reivich M, Jehle J, Sokoloff L, et al: Measurement of regional cerebral blood flow with antipyrine-^{14}C in awake cats. J Appl Physiol 27:296–300, 1969.

19. Sakurada O, Kennedy C, Jehle J, et al: Measurement of local cerebral blood flow with iodo(^{14}C)antipyrine. Am J Physiol 234:H59–66, 1978.

20. Ingvar DH, Philipson L: Distribution of cerebral blood flow in dominant hemisphere during motor ideation and motor performance. Ann Neurol 2:230–237, 1977.

21. Ingvar DH: Brain activation patterns revealed by measurements of regional cerebral blood flow. In Cognitive Components in Cerebral Event-related Potentials and Selective Attention Progress in Clinical Neurology, Vol 6, Desmedt JE (ed), Basel, S Karger, pp. 200–215, 1979.

22. Bailliart P: La pression artérielle dans les branches de l'artère centrale de la retine; nouvelle technique pour la determiner. Ann d'ocul 154:648, 1917.

23. Antin S, Karlan R: Ophthalmodynamometry. Neurology 12:153–156, 1962.

24. Baurmann M: Druckmessungen an der Netzhaut Zentralarterie. Ber ü d Versamml d deutsch opth Gesellsch 51:228, 1936.

25. Thomas MH, Petrohelos MA: Diagnostic significance of retinal artery pressure in internal carotid involvement. Am J Ophth 36:335–346, 1953.

26. Svien HJ, Hollenhorst RW: Pressure in retinal arteries after ligation or occlusion of the carotid artery. Proc Staff Meet Mayo Clin 31:684–692, 1956.

27. Hollenhorst RW: Discussion. Proceedings of Third Princeton Conference. In Cerebral Vascular Diseases, Millikan CH, Siekert RG, Whisnant JP (eds), New York, Grune & Stratton, p. 19, 1961.

28. Heyman A: Ophthalmoscopy–fluorescein appearance time. Proceedings of Third Princeton Conference. In Cerebral Vascular Diseases, Millikan CH, Siekert RG, Whisnant JP (eds), New York, Grune & Stratton, pp. 13–20, 1961.

29. Novotny HR, Alvis DL: A method of photographing fluorescence in circulating blood of the human eye. School of Aviation Medicine, USAF Aerospace Medical Center (ATC) Brooks Air Force Base, TX 60–82:1–4, (Sept) 1960.

30. Bynke HG, Krakau CET: A handy instrument for oculosphygmography with some clinical results. Ophthalmologica (Basel) 148:367–373, 1964.

31. Uyama M, Nakai H: Clinical studies on pulse wave of the cornea and retinal arterial pressure. Acta Soc Ophthal (Japan) 65:40, 1961.

32. Hager H: Die Diagnose der Karotisthrombose durch den Augenarzt. Klin Mbl Augenheilk 141:801, 1962.

33. Castren JA, Lavikainen P: New method of diagnosing carotid disease. Acta Ophthal 42:219–223, 1964.

34. Bynke HG: Screening diagnosis of carotid occlusion by means of oculosphygmography. Neurology 16:383–391, 1966.

35. Wood EH: Thermography in the diagnosis of cerebrovascular disease. Radiology 85:270–283, 1965.

36. Fields WS: Aortocranial occlusive vascular disease (stroke). Clin Symposia (Ciba) 26:3–31, 1974.

37. Lawrence C, Britton W, Still C: Ophthalmic pulse in carotid disease. Presented at the 22nd Clinical Meeting of the Wilmer Residents Assoc., April 26, 1963.

38. Brockenbrough EC, Lawrence C, Schwenk WG: Ocular plethysmography: A new technique for the evaluation of carotid obstructive disease. Rev Surg 24:299–302, 1967.

39. Best M, Pola R, Plechaty G, et al: Ocular pulse studies in carotid stenosis. Arch Ophthal 85:730–737, 1971.

40. Galin MA, Baras I, Best M, et al: Methods of suction ophthalmodyna-momometry. Ann Ophthal 1:439–443, 1970.

41. Gee W, Smith CA, Hinson CE, et al: Ocular pneumoplethysmography in carotid artery disease. Med Instrum 8:244–248, 1974.

42. Hays RJ, Levinson SA, Wylie EJ: Intra-operative measurement of carotid back pressure as a guide to operative management for carotid endarterectomy. Surg 72:953–960, 1972.

43. Kartchner MM, McRae LP: Auscultation for carotid bruits in cerebro-vascular insufficiency. JAMA 210:494–497, 1969.

44. Kartchner MM, McRae LP, Morrison FD: Noninvasive detection and evaluation of carotid occlusive disease. Arch Surg 106:528–535, 1973.

45. Doppler C: Über das farbige Licht der Doppelsterne und einiger anderer Gestirne des Himmels. Abh Kgl Böhm Ges Wissensch (Prag), pp. 465–482, 1842.

46. Müller HR: The diagnosis of internal carotid artery occlusion by direc-tional Doppler sonography of the ophthalmic artery. Neurology 22:816–823, 1972.

47. Franklin DL, Schlegel WA, Rushmer RF: Blood flow measured by Dop-pler frequency shift of back-scattered ultrasound. Science 134:564–565, 1961.

48. Miyazaki M, Kato K: Measurement of cerebral blood flow by ultrasonic Doppler technique. Hemodynamic comparisons of right and left carotid arteries in patients with hemiplegia. Jap Circ J 29:383, 1965.

49. Stegall HF, Rushmer RF, Baker DW: A transcutaneous ultrasonic blood velocity meter. J Appl Physiol 21:707–711, 1966.

50. Maroon JC, Pieroni DW, Campbell RL: Ophthalmosonometry, an ultra-sonic method for assessing carotid blood flow. J Neurosurg 30:238–246, 1969.

51. Thomas GI, Spencer MP, Jones TW, et al: Noninvasive carotid bifur-cation mapping. Am J Surg 128:168–174, 1974.

52. Reid JM, Spencer MP: Ultrasonic Doppler techniques for imaging blood vessels. Science 176:1235–1236, 1972.

53. Leopold GR: Pulse echo ultrasonography for the noninvasive imaging of vascular anatomy. In Noninvasive Diagnostic Techniques in Vascular Disease, Bernstein EF (ed), St. Louis, C.V. Mosby, pp. 219–228, 1985.

54. Kristensen JK, Eiken M, von Wowern F: Ultrasonic diagnosis of carotid artery disease. J Neurosurg 35:40–44, 1971.

55. Olinger C: Ultrasonic carotid echoarteriography. AJR 106:282–295, 1969.

56. Hertz CH: Ultrasonic engineering in heart diagnosis. Am J Cardiol 19:6–17, 1967.

57. Howry DH and Bliss WR: Ultrasonic visualization of soft tissue struc-tures of the body. J Lab Clin Med 40:579–592, 1952.

58. Blue SK, McKinney WM, Barnes R, et al: Ultrasonic B-mode scanning for study of extracranial vascular disease. Neurology 22:1079–1085, 1972.

59. Fields WS: Noninvasive testing for carotid artery disease. Texas Med 78:45–48, 1982.

60. Hokanson DE, Mozersky DJ, Sumner DS, et al: Ultrasonic arteriog-raphy: A new approach to arterial visualisation. Biomed Eng 6:420, 1971.

61. Sumner DS, Moore DJ, Miles RD: Doppler ultrasonic arteriography and flow velocity analysis in carotid artery disease. In Noninvasive Diagnostic Techniques in Vascular Disease, Bernstein EF (ed), St. Louis, C.V. Mosby, pp. 349–366, 1985.

62. Sumner DS, Strandness DE, Jr., Hokanson DE, et al: Pulsed-Doppler ultrasonic arteriography in the diagnosis of carotid arterial stenosis (abstract). Stroke 7:3, 1976.

63. Lusby RJ, Woodcock JP, Skidmore R, et al: Carotid artery disease: A prospective evaluation of pulsed Doppler imaging. Ultrasound Med & Biol 7:365–370, 1981.

64. Russell JB: Pulsed Doppler ultrasonic arteriography. In Noninvasive Diagnosis of Vascular Disease, Hershey FB, Barnes RW, Sumner DS (eds), Pasadena, Appleton Davies, pp. 268–280, 1984.

65. Hennerici M, Rautenberg W, Sitzer G, et al: Transcranial Doppler ultrasound for the assessment of intracranial arterial flow velocity—Part 1: Examination technique and normal values. Surg Neurol 27:439–448, 1987.

66. Aaslid R, Markwalder TM, Nornes H: Non-invasive transcranial Doppler ultrasound recording of flow velocity in basal cerebral arteries. J Neurosurg 57:769–774, 1982.

67. Aaslid R, Huber P, Nornes H: Evaluation of cerebrovascular spasm with transcranial Doppler ultrasound. J Neurosurg 60:37–41, 1984.

68. Seiler RW, Grolimund P, Aaslid R, et al: Cerebral vasospasm evaluated by transcranial ultrasound correlated with clinical grade and CT-visualized subarachnoid hemorrhage. J Neurosurg 64:594–600, 1986.

69. Blackshear WM, Jr., Phillips DJ, Thiele BL, et al: Detection of carotid occlusive disease by ultrasound imaging and pulsed Doppler spectrum analysis. Surgery 86:698–706, 1979.

70. Mercier LA, Greenleaf JF, Evans TC, Jr., et al: High resolution ultrasound arteriography: A comparison with carotid angiography. In Noninvasive Diagnostic Techniques in Vascular Disease, Bernstein EF (ed), St. Louis, C.V. Mosby, pp. 231–244, 1978.

71. Fell G, Phillips DJ, Chikos PM, et al: Ultrasonic duplex scanning for disease of the carotid artery. Circulation 64:1191–1195, 1981.

72. Bluth EI, Kay D, Merritt CRB, et al: Sonographic characterization of carotid plaque: Detection of hemorrhage. AJNR 7:311–315, 1986.

73. Imparato A, Riles T, Gorstein F: The carotid bifurcation plaque: Pathologic findings associated with cerebral ischemia. Stroke 10:238–244, 1979.

74. Imparato A, Riles T, Mintzer R, et al: The importance of hemorrhage in the relationship between gross morphologic characteristics and cerebral symptoms in 376 carotid artery plaques. Ann Surg 197:195–203, 1983.

75. Lusby R, Ferrell L, Ehrenfeld W, et al: Carotid plaque hemorrhage: Its role in production of cerebral ischemia. Arch Surg 117:1479–1488, 1982.

76. Lees RS, Kistler JP: Noninvasive diagnosis of extracranial cerebrovascular disease. Neurol Clin 2:667–675, 1984.

77. Oldendorf WH: Isolated flying spot detection of radiodensity discontin-

uities—displaying the internal structural pattern of a complex object. IRE Trans in Bio-med Electronics 8:68–72, 1961.

78. Hounsfield GN: Computerized transverse axial scanning (tomography): Part 1. Description of system. Br J Radiol 46:1016–1022, 1973.

79. New PFJ, Scott WR, Schnur JA, et al: Computerized axial tomography with the EMI scanner. Radiology 110:109–123, 1974.

80. Ambrose J: Computerized transverse axial scanning (tomography): Part 2. Clinical application. Br J Radiol 46:1023–1047, 1973.

81. Kistler JP, Hochberg FH, Brooks BR, et al: Computerized axial tomography: Clinicopathologic correlation. Neurology 25:201–209, 1975.

82. Campbell JK, Houser OW, Stevens JC, et al: Computed tomography and radionuclide imaging in the evaluation of ischemic stroke. Radiology 126:695–702, 1978.

83. Sandercock P, Molyneux A, Warlow C: Value of computed tomography in patients with stroke: Oxfordshire Community Stroke Project. Br Med J 290:193–197, 1985.

84. Kinkel WR, Jacobs L: Computerized axial transverse tomography in cerebrovascular disease. Neurology 26:924–930, 1976.

85. Frisén L, Lindberg B, Kjällman L, et al: Detection of extracranial carotid stenosis by computed tomography. Lancet 1:1319–1320, 1979.

86. Bloch F, Hanson WW, Packard ME: Nuclear induction. Physical Rev 69:127, 1946.

87. Purcell EM, Torry HC, Pound RV: Resonance absorption by nuclear magnetic moments in a solid. Physical Rev 69:37–38, 1946.

88. Reeves RC, Pohost GM: Nuclear magnetic resonance in vascular imaging. In Noninvasive Diagnostic Techniques in Vascular Disease, Bernstein EF (ed), St. Louis, C.V. Mosby, pp. 261–268, 1985.

89. Davis KR, Kistler JP, Buonanno FS: Clinical neuroimaging approaches to cerebrovascular diseases. Neurol Clin 2:655–665, 1984.

90. Kistler JP, Buonanno FS, DeWitt LD, et al: Vertebral basilar territory stroke: Delineation by proton nuclear magnetic resonance imaging. Stroke 15:417–426, 1984.

91. Ruszkowski JT, Damadian R, Hanafee W, et al: MR imaging carotid artery. Works in Progress, Neuroradiology Session, RSNA, Chicago, Nov. 19, 1985.

92. Budinger TF, Ganz E, Price DC, et al: Radionuclide and nuclear magnetic resonance techniques of evaluating atherosclerosis. In Clinical Diagnosis of Atherosclerosis: Quantitative Methods of Evaluation, Bond MG, Insull W, Jr., Glagov S, et al. (eds), New York, Springer-Verlag, pp. 189–219, 1982.

93. Macchi PJ, Grossman RI, Gomori JM, et al: High field MR imaging of cerebral venous thrombosis. JCAT 10:10–15, 1986.

94. Phelps ME, Hoffman EJ, Mullani NA, et al: Application of annihilation coincidence detection to transaxial reconstruction tomography. J Nucl Med 16:210–223, 1975.

95. Phelps ME, Hoffman EJ, Mullani NA, et al: Transaxial emission reconstruction tomography: Coincidence detection of positron-emitting radionuclides. In Noninvasive Brain Imaging, Radionuclides and Computed Tomography, DeBlanc H, Sorenson JA (eds), New York, Society of Nuclear Medicine, pp. 87–109, 1975.

96. Ter-Pogossian MM, Phelps ME, Hoffman EJ, et al: A positron emission transaxial tomograph for nuclear medicine imaging (PETT). Radiology 114:89–98, 1975.

97. Phelps ME, Mazziotta JC, Huang SC: Study of cerebral function with positron computed tomography. J Cereb Blood Flow Metab 2:113–162, 1982.

98. Correia JA, Alpert NM, Ackerman RH: Positron emission tomography (PET). In Noninvasive Diagnostic Techniques in Vascular Disease, Bernstein EF (ed), St. Louis, C.V. Mosby, pp. 250–260, 1985.

99. Kessler R: Discussion of application of PET systems. 33rd Annual Meeting of Society of Nuclear Medicine. Reported in Radiology Today 3:12, 1986.

100. Thakur ML, Welch MJ, Joist JH, et al: Indium-111 labeled platelets: Studies on preparation and evaluation of *in vitro* and *in vivo* functions. Thromb Res 9:345–357, 1976.

101. Davis HH, Heaton WA, Siegel BA, et al: Scintigraphic detection of atherosclerotic lesions and venous thrombi in man by indium-111-labeled autologous platelets. Lancet 1:1185–1187, 1978.

102. Finklestein S, Miller A, Callahan RJ, et al: Imaging of acute arterial injury with [111]indium labeled platelets: Comparison with scanning electron micrographs. Radiology 145:155–159, 1982.

103. Lees RS, Lees AM, Strauss HW: External imaging of human atherosclerosis. J Nucl Med 24:154–156, 1983.

7

Hypertension and Stroke

Hypertension is the most prevalent treatable risk factor for stroke, and it appears that this risk increases as blood pressure levels rise. Our present view of the significance of hypertension in the various stroke syndromes has an interesting background.

Primary Intracerebral Hemorrhage

Whisnant relates:

> More than 250 years ago in 1714, Cardinal Antonio Francisco Sanvitalis was seized with a violent pain in the head and a loss of power and feeling in the left part of his body, and he lay as if overcome with a profound sleep. After "blood was taken away . . . when the right jugular vein was opened by Valsalva's order, for about 4 hours after, his internal senses were awakened, and his speech, for more than an hour, was restored." The same change occurred on the following night "but this rousing was his last."[1]

This is Morgagni's account, published shortly after the event in the eighteenth century, concerning the treatment of "sanguineous apoplexy."[2] According to Russell:

> Hardening of the pulse in association with apoplexy was known long before blood pressure could be measured and was noted by Wepfer (1658)[4] in his original description of cerebral hemorrhage verified at autopsy. He saw the area of hemorrhage in the floor of the lateral ventricle, found that the small blood vessels were excessively fragile and looked without success for a ruptured artery or vein. Succeeding generations of pathologists have fared

little better and the one indisputable fact is the almost invariable association between cerebral hemorrhage and high blood pressure.[3]

Charcot and Bouchard (1868) first described an association between minute, or miliary, aneurysms of intracerebral arteries and parenchymal hemorrhage.[5,6] They dissected the brains of 84 patients dying of stroke and reported that three of the brains had small aneurysms within a massive intracerebral hemorrhage.[6] Small grape-like swellings were present in large numbers along many intracerebral arteries in these patients.[7]

Ellis (1909)[8] wrote that "the so-called miliary aneurysms of cerebral hemorrhage are false aneurysms . . . preceded by simple rupture or by dissecting aneurysms of the affected artery."[9] In 1910, Pick,[10] who introduced the method of shaking up the disorganized brain substance with saline in order to isolate the diseased vessels, stated that he was unable to demonstrate true miliary aneurysms as a cause of cerebral hemorrhage.[9] He showed that some of these swellings along a vessel were small perivascular hematomas and were a result rather than the cause of hemorrhage. The aneurysm theory was then discredited and other reasons for bleeding were presented.[7] Ellis also quoted Osler (1905) as saying that "we must conclude that spontaneous rupture (of diseased arteries) may occur without the previous formation of aneurysms,"[11] and himself stated that aneurysm formation is not an essential preliminary to the occurrence of cerebral hemorrhage.

These statements are in agreement with textbooks of pathology during the 1920s. The prevalent view was that miliary aneurysms of the intracerebral arteries are a rarity, and some authors expressed doubt as to whether they actually occur.[9] The "miliary aneurysms" to which we are referring are those confined to the small parenchymal arteries; not those aneurysms which are found on the larger branches of the circle of Willis and which may rupture, causing spontaneous subarachnoid hemorrhage.

Green (1930)[9] showed that small, but definite, aneurysms do occur and may be a source of bleeding.[7] He found 3 aneurysms in a painstaking histologic examination of 10 brains from hypertensive subjects. His method was to take multiple blocks of tissue and inspect serial sections under the microscope; the few lesions found attest to the limitations of this method.[12] Green also suggested that miliary aneurysms arise only where atheromatous change involves the media of an artery to an extreme degree. Russell (1963)[3] used postmortem X-ray microangiography following barium injection to survey 54 brains and described many more aneurysms, particularly in elderly hypertensive subjects.[12]

Both Russell[3] and Cole and Yates (1967)[12] studied aneurysms in hypertensive and normotensive patients at autopsy. Russell found aneurysms in 93% of patients with diastolic blood pressures over 110 mm Hg and in only 28.5% of normotensives. Cole and Yates also found many more aneurysms in the hypertensive group (46% of patients) than in the normotensive group (7%). In the latter group, aneurysms were found exclusively in the elderly (over 65 years).

Cole and Yates summarized:

> . . . as hypertension can be adequately controlled in many cases, such [intracerebral] hemorrhage is, to a large extent, a preventable disease. . . . We have no evidence as to how long hypertension must be present before aneurysms appear, or of the fate of the lesions if the blood pressure is reduced to normal levels.[12]

They also believed that their study added support to the view that the administration of anticoagulants to hypertensives is hazardous.

Both cerebral hemorrhage and cerebral aneurysms are disorders of middle-aged and elderly hypertensive persons.[7] The aneurysms, or swellings along the vessels, cannot be the result of cerebral hemorrhage (as stated by Pick) since they are present in hypertensive and normotensive brains in the absence of bleeding.[3] As Russell wrote:

> The combination of age and hypertension produces a degeneration of muscular and elastic element of small cerebral arteries which goes on to the formation of multiple miliary aneurysms, especially in the basal ganglia.[3]

However, elderly hypertensive persons do not appear to develop aneurysms in other microcirculatory beds throughout the body.[13] This may be explained by the fact that the small cerebral arteries are not only thin-walled, but, as shown by Gimbert (1865)[14] and confirmed by Clarke (1965),[15] they have no vasa vasorum.[16]

Hypertension and Atherosclerosis

Although atherosclerosis of blood vessels was recognized as early as around 1500, Francois Bayle (1677)[17] was among the first to describe calcification and plaques in the cerebral arteries and relate these to apoplexy.[18] When Wepfer (1658) wrote that those most liable to apoplexy were the obese, those whose face and hands were livid, and those whose pulse is constantly unequal, he may have been the first to infer that hypertensive persons or patients with cardiac disease are more susceptible to strokes.[4,18]

The early landmark publications (prior to 1915) establishing cause and effect relationships among atherosclerosis, embolism, and strokes have been reviewed in Chapter 1. The recognition that hypertension is an important risk factor for stroke developed during a more recent period. Such a relationship could become apparent only after the invention of a sphygmomanometer that could be operated without breaking the skin and thereby become widely utilized by physicians. Samuel Siegfried von Basch invented such a device and published a description in 1881. However, his machine was inaccurate and soon abandoned. An Italian physician, Scipione Riva-Rocci (Figure 7.1), created the prototype of today's instrument in 1896. His product measured only systolic pressure, but in 1905, Nikolai Korotkoff, using a stethoscope, derived the technique for recording diastolic pressure.[19]

During the 1920s, articles suggesting a kinship between hypertension and atherosclerosis in cardiac disease, as well as articles on treatment of essential hypertension, began appearing in medical journals. In 1930,

Figure 7.1. SCIPIONE RIVA-ROCCI
(From Triangle—The Sandoz Journal of Medical Science 6(3):73, 1963. Courtesy of Sandoz Ltd., Basel, Switzerland)

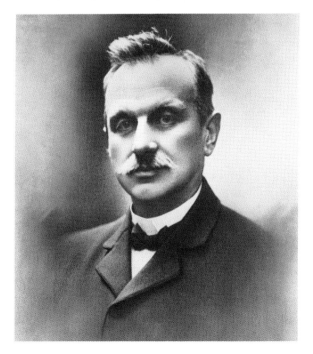

Schwartz[20] wrote of apoplectic complications of essential hypertension, and Goldringer[21] related increased blood pressure and tonus of arteries to cerebral hemorrhage. Gunewardene (1932) stated that strokes often attributed to other factors, such as shock, exertion, and emotion, are the result of already existing high arterial pressure exacerbated by the influence of these factors.[22]

By the 1950s, atherosclerosis at various body sites was under intense investigation by researchers worldwide. Fisher (1964) stated:

> Arterial hypertension alters the distribution of atheroma by leading in some cases to its deposition in the smaller vessels over the surface of the cerebral hemispheres, cerebellar lobes, and in the penetrating branches of the cerebral arteries. The presence of atheroma in the surface arteries over the hemisphere bespeaks hypertension. . . . Not only does hypertension change the distribution of atheroma, but it clearly and unequivocally aggravates the process at all sites.[23]

In 1965, Berkson and Stamler reported their epidemiologic findings on cerebrovascular disease and wrote that their most conclusive observation was the striking relationship between hypertensive disease and strokes; the two disorders paralleled each other in morbidity, mortality, and racial incidence.[24] They also found that preexistent cardiac disease or electrocardiogram abnormalities predispose to a high rate of future cerebrovascular disease.

Robertson and Strong (1968) in addition to stating that persons with high blood pressure are more prone to develop cerebrovascular disease than normotensives also believed that the serum lipids in hypertensives differ from normal in such a way as to cause a greater severity of atherosclerosis.[25] They cited certain racial groups with a high overall level of atherosclerosis, in whom hypertension apparently added to the risk of mortality by aggravating the mural arterial lesions at all stages. Robertson and Strong recounted:

> Hypertension and diabetes do not appear to be a primary cause of atherosclerosis because atherosclerosis may be severe and extensive in persons without either disease. However, when hypertension and diabetes are present, they accelerate the natural progression of atherosclerosis in all populations.[25]

Publications from the Framingham Study have been truly landmark articles, and, in 1970, Kannel et al. wrote:

> The exact mechanism of hypertension in the occurrence of strokes is incompletely understood. That it accelerates atherosclerosis in the cerebral

arteries is not well established. That it may mechanically damage vessels seems likely. An indirect influence precipitating strokes by impaired cardiac function leading to reduced cerebral perfusion in the region of severely narrowed vessels also seems likely. . . . Hypertension associated with evidence of cardiac involvement is clearly more ominous.

The evidence for a predominant role of hypertension in accelerating cerebral atherogenesis is disappointingly weak. The preponderance of evidence seems to emphasize a multifactorial causation of atherosclerosis, but if a single common denominator does exist, then some aberration of the metabolism or transport of lipid must be regarded as the chief contender.[26]

In the Framingham population, asymptomatic hypertension was associated with a risk of atherothrombotic brain infarction about four times that of normotensives.

Systolic blood pressure correlates more closely with the risk of cerebral infarction than does diastolic blood pressure, although most trials have concentrated on the latter.[27] Two studies of older persons have shown that hypertension is a risk factor for subsequent stroke among persons having some target-organ damage (heart disease, TIAs, intermittent claudication, electrocardiogram abnormalities), but not among those without damage.[28,29]

Atherothrombotic brain infarction is the most common type of stroke, accounting for 57% of all strokes. Fifteen percent are secondary to cerebral embolus; 16% result from intracranial hemorrhage (2/3 subarachnoid and 1/3 intracerebral); TIA only and stroke due to other causes are 6% each.[30] The most influential contributor to thrombotic infarction, other than age, is high systolic blood pressure, and this is true in both sexes.[30]

Hypertensive Encephalopathy

In 1871, Traube wrote of acute edema of the brain, which he regarded as a consequence of decreased blood protein and increased arterial pressure.[31,32] He believed that either of these factors could increase passage of fluid out of the vessels into brain substance and precipitate a cerebral attack.[32] In his time, Traube had no way of measuring either factor. No clear evidence has since been produced to show that plasma protein has any role in this disorder.[32] Traube also believed that defective constriction of cerebral arteries occurred. Allbutt (1895)[33] stated that for some hypertensive patients the outlook was good for many years.[34]

As the recognition of cases increased in number and as the use of the

Riva-Rocci sphygmomanometer became general, physicians gradually realized that there were variations in the severity of the condition. This led Volhard and Fahr (1914)[35] and Volhard (1931)[36] to write of benign and malignant forms of hypertension.[34] Also, in the early years of the present century, any acute cerebral symptoms in the hypertensive patient which could not be ascribed to a definite stroke were generally regarded as the result of renal failure.[37] These episodes were included in the symptom complex of uremia, and Volhard and Fahr first clearly distinguished them from true uremia. They termed them "pseudouremia" and found that hypertension was invariable in the attacks. Volhard (Figure 7.2) considered cerebral arterioles to be more constricted than arterioles elsewhere, so that cerebral blood flow became diminished and capillaries were damaged by anoxia, allowing fluid and protein to pass out into brain parenchyma.[32] However, Pickering (1948) provided information that cerebral arterioles do not constrict more strongly to a constrictor substance than arterioles elsewhere; in fact, the reverse is true.[32]

Oppenheimer and Fishberg (1928) first used the term "hypertensive encephalopathy."[38] They wrote:

> It has become clear that these cerebral symptoms are correlated with hypertension, being a manifestation of circulatory disturbances in the brain consequent on the hypertension. For this reason, we have termed the cerebral syndrome the hypertensive encephalopathy. . . .
>
> These cerebral episodes occur only in patients with arterial hypertension and are generally preceded by an additional rise in blood pressure above the previous high level. . . . Available evidence indicates strongly that the hypertensive encephalopathy is the result of cerebral anemia produced by cerebral vasoconstriction. The cerebral edema which is present in some, but not in all, of the cases is secondary to the vasoconstriction, though the exact mechanism of the connection is not clear.[38]

Pickering stated that hypertensive encephalopathy comprises two distinct clinical and pathologic conditions. In acute hypertension (and chronic hypertension with recent exacerbation), attacks of headache, vomiting, convulsions, and coma are generally due to acute edema of the brain. In chronic hypertension, there are attacks of sensory or motor paralysis of brief duration, a tendency to complete resolution, and usually, the maintenance of consciousness.[32] Today, episodes of this latter type might be termed lacunar infarcts or TIAs. These attacks were attributed to spasm of a cerebral artery by Peabody in 1891.[39] He observed a 56-year-old man with six transient episodes of right hemiparesis in whom neither a cerebral infarct nor complete occlusion of a cerebral artery was found postmortem,

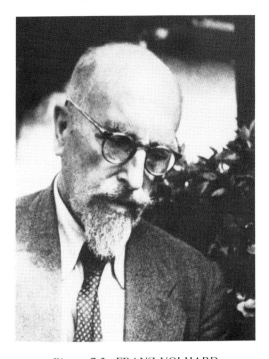

Figure 7.2. FRANZ VOLHARD

(From MacMahon HE: Malignant nephrosclerosis—50 years later. Journal of the History of Medicine and Allied Sciences 21:125–146, 1966, with permission from Yale Medical Library, New Haven, CT, copyright 1966)

although the middle cerebral and other arteries were grossly atheromatous. Volhard wrote that vasospasm did occur elsewhere and used intermittent claudication and angina as examples. Osler wrote of the cerebral complications of Reynaud's disease.[40,41] Pickering believed that the attacks in chronic hypertension were probably not due to cerebral arterial spasm but to sudden organic arterial occlusion, for example, by a thrombus.

Data in favor of the spasm theory to explain attacks of acute hypertension were provided by Byrom's classical studies of cerebral symptoms in rats with renal hypertension.[37,42–44] Events occurred only in animals with systolic pressures over 200 mm Hg.[45] He observed widespread intense vascular spasm by looking through a plastic cover over the brains of the rats; they suffered seizures and coma which were interpreted as being the counterpart of hypertensive encephalopathy.[46] There was diffuse and focal vasoconstriction, which corresponds with Volhard's concept of the process being primarily vasoconstrictive with generalized cerebral ischemia that goes on to focal and then diffuse cerebral edema.[45]

Byrom (1954) stated that this syndrome presents to the clinician in many different patterns—generalized convulsions, local disturbances of cerebral function, and symptoms of increased intracranial pressure.[37] His evidence from rats with serious experimental renal hypertension suggested two grades of severity. In the first, underlying vasoconstriction is diffuse and controlled so that distribution of blood to tissues remains essentially normal (except when locally impeded by atheroma); in the second, there is superimposed on physiologic vasoconstriction a state of focal but widespread pathologic spasm, which is a direct response to the strain of excessive intra-arterial pressure. This occurrence is a "simple physiological property of arterial muscle, namely, its faculty of contracting against a filling tension. . . . The arterial spasm which underlies these various changes can be abolished by removing its cause, i.e., by lowering the blood pressure."[37]

Lacunes

This word is from the Latin *lacuna*, "a hole or small cavity."[47] Following Dechambre's description and use of the word in 1838[48] (see Chapter 1), it appears that the next publication to include this term was Durand-Fardel's treatise (1843) on softening of the brain.[49] The pathologic findings in his Case #78 were:

> The striatum on each side showed a certain number of small lacunes with no associated alteration of color or consistency from whose surface there extended a fine meshwork containing very small vessels.[50]

The literature over the next 60 years contained very few references to lacunes. Proust (1866)[51] stated, "These cavities which have received the name lacunes are usually no larger than a lentil or small pea."[50] Landouzy (1877)[52] called attention to a "hemorrhagic lacunar scar" in the centrum semiovale.[50] Raymond (1885)[53] described small cerebral lesions in elderly patients dying of uremia, but in his opinion the paralysis did not seem to be the result of such lacunes but due to an associated cerebral edema.[50] Comte (1900)[54] in his monograph on pseudobulbar paralysis referred to lacunes either by name or by description in 9 of the 11 cases studied.[50]

The first researchers to characterize the lesion clearly and to present the principal aspects of the clinical situation were Marie and Ferrand.

Marie (Figure 7.3), in whose laboratory Ferrand worked, gave a paper[55] in 1901, which was an abbreviated version of Ferrand's monograph[56] which appeared in 1902.[50] Marie found lacunes in 45 out of 50 brains examined at autopsy and recognized the small cavity as a healed infarct resulting from "rupture or obliteration" of a perforating artery or its branches due to local arteriosclerosis.[50] During life, the patients had usually had a sudden hemiparesis with good recovery or an acute clumsiness of an extremity; pseudobulbar palsy was common.[50] Marie first used the expression "état lacunaire" in diagnosing persons affected by multiple lacunes[57] and stressed that lacunes, rather than hemorrhage or infarction, were more often the cause of hemiparesis in the elderly.[47] Marie wrote:

> . . . the patient advances slowly with a shuffling gait. There is no spasticity but a rather soft movement. Each step is only 10–15 cm in length

Figure 7.3. PIERRE MARIE
(From Rolleston H: Medical eponyms. Annals of Medical History 9:1–12, 1937. Photograph from the author's *The Endocrine Organs in Health and Disease,* with permission from Oxford University Press)

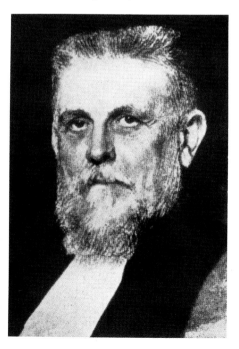

and the lower extremities are maintained in slightly flexed position with the trunk bent forward.[47]

The marked difficulty in walking is not relevant to the severity of the motor deficit, which is usually of a much more minor degree. Dejerine (1914) used the phrase "marche à petite pas."[58] (These descriptions are also typical of the festinating gait seen in paralysis agitans.) Dementia can be a prominent feature of lacunar disease, although it may not occur at all, and the degree of dementia does not seem to correlate with the number or site of lacunes.[59,60] Some patients with multiple lacunes present the typical triad of gait disturbance, dementia, and incontinence characteristic of normal–pressure hydrocephalus.[61–63] The bilateral lesions resulting in pseudobulbar palsy are often lacunar in nature, and "lacunar paraplegia" was first delineated in 1905 by Lejonne and Lhermitte.[64,47]

If a patient has a gradual loss of cognition without episodic events, which are the hallmark of significant occlusive cerebrovascular disease, there is no justification for making a diagnosis of lacunar disease or of atherosclerotic dementia, as is often done.[65] However, Fisher has described episodic deficits that are correlated pathologically with lacunes deep within the brain substance. He has identified four syndromes: pure motor hemiplegia,[66] pure sensory stroke,[67] crural paresis with homolateral ataxia,[68] and dysarthria with clumsiness of one hand.[69] The circumscribed nature of the focal neurologic deficit, a stuttering onset, and clearing in days to weeks are listed as diagnostic criteria. Fisher has concluded that these lesions occur on small penetrating branches of intracranial arteries because of hypertension.[65]

Hughes et al. (1954) reported 51 patients with chronic arterial hypertension with personality changes and pseudobulbar palsy.[70] In 15 studied at autopsy, there were multiple lacunes. The authors suggested as the cause of the infarcts, eddying in the stem of the middle cerebral artery interfering with flow to the penetrating branches.[50] However, it was Fisher (1965) who first emphasized the role of hypertension and atherosclerosis in the pathogenesis of état lacunaire.[50] In a series of 1042 consecutive adults whose brains were removed at autopsy, 11% had one or more lacunes.[50]

Also, Fisher (1969) appears to be the first to clearly establish the underlying cause of lacunes.[71] By meticulously examining serial sections, he showed that vascular occlusion actually accounted for the infarct seen in the neighboring tissue. The lacune and the responsible arterial occlusion rarely lay in the same plane, and when arterial disorganization was found adjacent to a lacune in the same section, the two were usually unrelated.

Antihypertensive Drugs and Prevention of Stroke

With malignant hypertension, there was early evidence of the capacity of hypotensive drugs to prolong life.[72] Keith et al. (1939)[73] showed that without treatment about 79% of patients with this disorder were dead within one year after diagnosis, whereas Dunstan and colleagues (1958)[74] found that among 84 patients receiving treatment at least 50% survived three years. These latter authors stated, "Survival is improved in patients who undertake treatment before malignant hypertension has caused extensive vascular damage."[74]

However, trials that assessed the role of essential hypertension of a more moderate degree in the occurrence of stroke (either atherothrombotic or hemorrhagic) took longer to achieve meaningful findings. Although Pierson and Hoobler (1957)[75,76] reported that a reduction in diastolic blood pressure of 20 mm Hg following sympathectomy in patients with hypertension and stroke reduced the annual stroke occurrence from 6% to less than 1%,[76] it wasn't until the 1960s that articles on trials of hypertensive drugs to avert strokes began appearing in medical journals. The early studies were not controlled but simply compared a treated group of hypertensive patients with another group from a previous time or with a group of patients who had refused treatment.[77]

An effort of such design was conducted by Leishman (1963) in persons with initial diastolic blood pressures above 120 mm Hg.[72] Drug treatment appeared to result in a distinct fall in three- to five-year mortality rates; in subjects with diastolic blood pressures above 130 mm Hg, the reduction was largely due to prevention of cerebral hemorrhage and renal failure. The author reported that the fatal strokes that did occur among treated individuals possibly reflected the presence of cerebral atherosclerosis rather than hypertension.

Marshall (1964) stated:

> . . . there has been considerable reluctance to prescribe long-term hypotensive therapy for patients who, after recovery from a cerebrovascular accident, are found to be hypertensive. This reluctance stems from the fear that hypotension may precipitate further cerebrovascular ischemic episodes.[78]

He treated 39 such patients (with diastolic blood pressures of 110 mm Hg or higher) for three years, while following 42 untreated subjects as a control group. He used long-term hypotensive therapy and demonstrated that 90% of the treated group versus 66% of the untreated group were alive after three years. The incidence of further stroke in men was significantly less in the treated group; in women, the difference did not quite reach significance.

Hamilton et al. (1964) in the first prospective trial studied persons with asymptomatic hypertension.[79] All subjects were under 60 years, and none had signs or symptoms of any arterial disease. All had a sustained diastolic pressure of at least 110 mm Hg, but all denied angina, claudication, or TIAs. All had palpable carotid and foot pulses, no bruit over carotid or femoral vessels, no electrocardiogram changes to suggest myocardial infarction. Among 10 men treated with hypotensive therapy for 2 to 6 years, none suffered a stroke. Among 12 untreated men, 4 had strokes (1 a fatal cerebral hemorrhage), 1 had a myocardial infarction, 1 had severe headaches requiring hypotensive therapy, and 2 had signs of left ventricular hypertrophy. Thus, 8 of 12 untreated men showed complications of hypertension.[76] The difference between treated and untreated patients was highly significant.

Among women, hypertension was more difficult to control. There was no difference in outcomes between the total groups of treated and untreated women. However, among those in whom adequate control of hypertension was achieved, there were no strokes and only one complication.[76]

The Veterans Administration Cooperative Study (1967)[80] and (1970)[81] was a prospective, randomized, double-blind trial involving 523 men with initial diastolic blood pressures in the range of 90 to 130 mm Hg. There were 143 patients whose initial diastolic pressures were 115 to 129 mm Hg, but the trial was terminated after an average follow-up of only 18 months in this subgroup because of a highly significant difference in morbid events in the control group as compared with treated persons.[77] Twenty-seven severe, complicating events developed among placebo patients as compared with 2 in the treated group. Stroke occurred in 5 of the control patients and in 1 treated patient.

The remaining 380 men whose diastolic blood pressures ranged from 90 to 114 mm Hg were observed for an average follow-up of 3.3 years. Incidence of stroke was 20 in the control group and 5 in the treated group. When both subgroups were combined, cerebral hemorrhage was diagnosed in 4 and subarachnoid hemorrhage in 2 control patients. No hemorrhagic strokes were diagnosed among treated patients. These results suggested that antihypertensive drug therapy was more effective in preventing hemorrhagic than in preventing atherothrombotic stroke. Effectiveness was demonstrated at all ages.[77]

The National Heart Foundation of Australia studied patients with mild hypertension from 1973 to 1979.[82] A controlled trial of antihypertensive therapy in 3427 men and women with diastolic blood pressures from 95 to 109 mm Hg and systolic pressures less than 200 mm Hg was conducted. They were given either active treatment or placebo and followed for an average of four years. There was significant reduction in mortality in the treated group, mainly due to a reduction by two-thirds in deaths from cardiovascular disease. There were also fewer cerebrovascular events in the treated group. The incidence of TIAs, fatal stroke, and nonfatal stroke was reduced by 50% in the "on treatment" group.

Evans (1983) wrote:

> There is no doubt that at ages under 60 there is a positive association between blood pressure and risk of cerebrovascular stroke.[83]

In that age group, stroke is comparatively rare; only about 20% of strokes occur at ages under 60. We know less about the significance of high blood pressure at older ages when stroke is common. Three small studies on the relationship between blood pressure and stroke in the elderly failed to detect any statistically significant effect of blood pressure on stroke incidence or on mortality rates from all causes.[84−86]

Evans followed 2800 persons (age 65 and over) living in a geographically defined community. Subjects were visited regularly at home, where blood pressures were taken, and individuals were observed for strokes over a four-year period. There were 140 stroke events with slightly greater rates in males compared with females. He was unable to demonstrate any relationship between blood pressure and subsequent stroke in either sex. Therefore, he believes that prevention of stroke by screening the elderly with a single blood pressure reading is unlikely to be profitable.

Evans concluded:

> . . . our approach to stroke prevention in old age may need to be different from that employed in young adults. In the latter we may profitably remove causes such as high blood pressure but at older ages we should be attempting to interrupt mechanisms rather than attempting to remove causes which have already many years before initiated their baneful effects. It may therefore prove that antiplatelet agents will be more useful in preventing stroke in the old than the hypotensive drugs which are of benefit to the young.[83]

References

1. Whisnant JP: Medical therapy for primary intracerebral hemorrhage. Proceedings of Sixth Princeton Conference. In Cerebral Vascular Diseases, Toole JF, Siekert RG, Whisnant JP (eds), New York, Grune & Stratton, pp. 167–178, 1968.

2. Morgagni JB: Letter the second (translated by B. Alexander). In The Seats and Causes of Diseases. Vol. 1. London, A. Millar and T. Cadell, pp. 17–34, 1769.

3. Russell RWR: Observations on intracerebral aneurysms. Brain 86:425–442, 1963.

4. Wepfer JJ: Observationes Anatomicae, ex Cadaveribus Eorum, quos Sustulit Apoplexia, cum Exercitatione de Ejus Loco Affecto. Schaffhausen, Joh. Caspari Suteri, 1658. English translation in Baglivi G: The Practice of Physick. London, p. 461, 1704.

5. Charcot JM, Bouchard C: Nouvelles recherches sur la pathogénie de l'hémorrhagie cérèbrale. Arch Physiol Norm Path 1:110–127; 643–645; 725–734, 1868.

6. Santos-Buch CA, Goodhue WW, Ewald BH: Experimental production of miliary aneurysms with hypertension. Proceedings of Ninth Princeton Conference. In Cerebral Vascular Diseases, Whisnant JP, Sandok BA (eds), New York, Grune & Stratton, pp. 91–103, 1974.

7. Russell RWR: Pathogenesis of primary intracerebral hemorrhage. Proceedings of Sixth Princeton Conference. In Cerebral Vascular Diseases, Toole JF, Siekert RG, Whisnant JP (eds), New York, Grune & Stratton, pp. 152–160, 1968.

8. Ellis AG: The pathogenesis of spontaneous cerebral hemorrhage. Trans Path Soc Philadelphia 12:197–235, 1909.

9. Green FHK: Miliary aneurysms in the brain. J Path Bact 33:71–77, 1930.

10. Pick L: Über die sogenannten miliaren Aneurysmen der Hirngfässe. Berlin Klin Wochenschr 47:325–340, 1910.

11. Osler W: Practice of Medicine, 6th ed., p. 967, 1905.

12. Cole FM, Yates PO: The occurrence and significance of intracerebral microaneurysms. J Path Bact 93:393–411, 1967.

13. Schwartz CJ: Discussion. Proceedings of Sixth Princeton Conference. In Cerebral Vascular Diseases, Toole JF, Siekert RG, Whisnant JP (eds), New York, Grune & Stratton, p. 158, 1968.

14. Gimbert JL: Structure et texture des artères. Thèse No. 81, Paris, 1865.

15. Clarke JA: An x-ray microscopic study of the vasa vasorum of the intracranial arteries. Z Anat Entwicklungsgesch 124:396–400, 1965.

16. Elliott FA: Discussion. Proceedings of Sixth Princeton Conference. In Cerebral Vascular Diseases, Toole JF, Siekert RG, Whisnant JP (eds), New York, Grune & Stratton, p. 158, 1968.

17. Bayle F: Tractatus de Apoplexia. Toulouse, B. Guillemette, 1677.

18. Garrison FH: History of Neurology. Revised & enlarged by McHenry LC, Jr., Springfield, IL, Charles C Thomas, 1969.

19. McGrew RE: Encyclopedia of Medical History. New York, McGraw-Hill, p. 317, 1985.

20. Schwartz P: Apoplectic complications of essential hypertension. Nervenarzt 3:450–462, 1930.

21. Goldringer E: Über die Arteriellen Zeichen cerebraler Herde und ihre Wertung. Zeitschr für die gesamte Neurologie und Psychiatrie 124:820–828, 1930.

22. Gunewardene HO: The stroke in high arterial pressure. Brit Med J 1:180–182, 1932.

23. Fisher CM: Discussion. Proceedings of Fourth Princeton Conference. In Cerebral Vascular Diseases, Millikan CH, Siekert RG, Whisnant JP (eds), New York, Grune & Stratton, p. 172, 1964.

24. Berkson DM, Stamler J: Epidemiological findings in cerebrovascular diseases and their complications. J Atherosclerosis Res 5:189–202, 1965.

25. Robertson WB, Strong JP: Atherosclerosis in persons with hypertension and diabetes. Lab Invest 18:538–551, 1968.

26. Kannel WB, Wolf PA, Verter J, et al: Epidemiologic assessment of the role of blood pressure in stroke. The Framingham Study. JAMA 214:301–310, 1970.

27. Warlow C: Medical management. In Transient Ischemic Attacks, Warlow C, Morris PJ (eds), New York, Marcel Dekker, pp. 221–252, 1982.

28. Ostfeld AM, Shekelle RB, Klawans H, et al: Epidemiology of stroke in an elderly welfare population. Am J Public Health 64:450–458, 1974.

29. The American-Canadian Cooperative Study Group: Persantine aspirin trial in cerebral ischemia. Part III: Risk factors for stroke. Stroke 17:12–18, 1986.

30. Wolf PA: Hypertension as a risk factor for stroke. Proceedings of Ninth Princeton Conference. In Cerebral Vascular Diseases, Whisnant JP, Sandok BA (eds), New York, Grune & Stratton, pp. 105–112, 1974.

31. Traube L: Gesammelte Beitrage zur Pathologie und Physiologie. Vol. 2. Berlin, A. Hirschwald, p. 551, 1871.

32. Pickering GW: Transient cerebral paralysis in hypertension and in cerebral embolism with special reference to the pathogenesis of chronic hypertensive encephalopathy. JAMA 137:423–430, 1948.

33. Allbutt TC: Senile plethora or high arterial pressure in elderly persons. Abstr Trans Hunterian Soc, p. 35, 1896.

34. Keith NM, Wagener HP, Barker NW: Some different types of essential hypertension: Their course and prognosis. Am J Med Sci 197:332–343, 1939.

35. Volhard F, Fahr KT: Die Brightache Nierenkrankheit: Klinik Pathologie und Atlas. Berlin, Julius Springer, 8, p. 292, 1914.

36. Volhard F: Handbuch d. inn. Med. Berlin, 2nd ed., i, 1931.

37. Byrom FB: The pathogenesis of hypertensive encephalopathy and its relation to the malignant phase of hypertension. Experimental evidence from the hypertensive rat. Lancet 2:201–211, 1954.

38. Oppenheimer BS, Fishberg AM: Hypertensive encephalopathy. Arch Int Med 41:264–278, 1928.

39. Peabody GL: Relation between arterial disease and visceral changes. Tr Assoc Am Physicians 6:154, 1891.

40. Osler W: The cerebral complications of Reynaud's disease. Am J Med Sci 112:522–529, 1896.

41. Osler W: Reynaud's disease. Canad M A J 1:919, 1911.

42. Byrom FB, Dodson LF: Causation of acute arterial necrosis in hypertensive disease. J Path Bact 60:357–368, 1948.

43. Byrom FB, Dodson LF: The mechanism of the vicious circle in chronic hypertension. Clin Sci 8:1–10, 1949.

44. Byrom FB: The nature of malignancy in hypertensive disease. Lancet 1:516–520, 1963.

45. Corcoran AC: Relationship of hypertension to cerebral vascular disease. Proceedings of Second Princeton Conference. In Cerebral Vascular Diseases, Wright IS, Millikan CH (eds), New York, Grune & Stratton, pp. 68–80, 1957.

46. Page IH: Hypertension and its effect on the cerebral circulation. Proceedings of First Princeton Conference. In Cerebral Vascular Diseases, Wright IS, Luckey EH (eds), New York, Grune & Stratton, pp. 59–70, 1954.

47. Román GC: Lacunar dementia. In Senile Dementia of the Alzheimer Type. New York, Alan R. Liss, pp. 131–151, 1985.

48. Dechambre A: Mémoire sur la curabilité du ramollissement cérébral. Gaz Méd Paris 6:305–314, 1838.

49. Durand-Fardel M: Traité due ramollissement du cerveau. Paris, J. B. Baillière, 1843.

50. Fisher CM: Lacunes: Small, deep cerebral infarcts. Neurology 15:774–784, 1965.

51. Proust A: Des Différentes Formes de Ramollissement du Cerveau. Thèse d'aggrégation-Médicine, Paris, 1866.

52. Landouzy L: Case report. Hémeplégia droite—contracture tardive et atrophie musculaire des membres droits. Prog Méd (Paris) 5:992, 1877.

53. Raymond F: Sur la pathogenie de certains accidents paralytiques observes chez des vieillards. Rev Med 5:705, 1885.

54. Comte A: Des Paralysies Pseudo-Bulbaires. Thèse, Paris, Steinheil G (ed), 1900.

55. Marie P: Des foyers lacunaires de désintégration et de différents autres états cavitaires du cerveau. Rev Med 21:281–298, 1901.

56. Ferrand J: Essai sur l'hémiplégie des Vieillards. Les lacunes de désintégration cérébrale. Thèse, Paris, Rousset J (ed), 1902.

57. Gautier JC: Cerebral ischemia in hypertension. In Vascular Disease of the Central Nervous System, Russell RWR (ed), Edinburgh, Churchill Livingstone, pp. 224–244, 1983.

58. Dejerine J: Séméiologie des Affections du Système Nerveux. Paris, Masson et Cie, 1914.

59. Román GC: Les Lacunes Cérébrales: Étude Clinique et Neuropathologique

de 100 cas. Mémoire pour le Titre d'Assistant Étranger. Service de Neurologie et Neuropsychologie, Hôpital de la Salpêtrière, Université de Paris, France, 1975.

60. Román GC: Lagunas cerebrales. Estudio clínico y neuropatológico de 100 casos fatales. Rev Fac Med UN Colombia 39:115–125, 1981.

61. Hakim S, Adams RD: The special clinical problem of symptomatic hydrocephalus with normal cerebrospinal fluid pressure. Observations on cerebrospinal fluid hydrodynamics. J Neurol Sci 2:307–327, 1965.

62. Adams RD, Fisher CM, Hakim S, et al: Symptomatic occult hydrocephalus with "normal" cerebrospinal-fluid pressure. A treatable syndrome. N Engl J Med 273:117–126, 1965.

63. Katzman R: Normal pressure hydrocephalus. In Dementia, 2nd ed., Wells CE (ed), Philadelphia, F. A. Davis, pp. 69–92, 1977.

64. Lejonne P, Lhermitte J: Les paraplégies d'origine lacunaire et myelopathique chez le vieillard. Arch Gen Med 2:3009–3027; 3072–3986, 1905.

65. Kannel WB: Current status of the epidemiology of brain infarction associated with occlusive arterial disease. Stroke 2:295–318, 1971.

66. Fisher CM, Curry HB: Pure motor hemiplegia of vascular origin. Arch Neurol 13:30–44, 1965.

67. Fisher CM: Pure sensory stroke involving face, arm and leg. Neurology 15:76–80, 1965.

68. Fisher CM, Cole M: Homolateral ataxia and crural paresis: A vascular syndrome. J Neurol Neurosurg Psychiat 28:48–55, 1965.

69. Fisher CM: A lacunar stroke. The dysarthria-clumsy hand syndrome. Neurology 17:614–617, 1967.

70. Hughes W, Dodgson MCH, MacLennan DC: Chronic cerebral hypertensive disease. Lancet 2:770–774, 1954.

71. Fisher CM: The arterial lesions underlying lacunes. Acta Neuropath (Berlin) 12:1–15, 1969.

72. Leishman AWD: Merits of reducing high blood pressure. Lancet 1:1284–1288, 1963.

73. Keith NM, Wagener HP, Barker NW: Some different types of essential hypertension: Their course and prognosis. Am J Med Sci 197:332–343, 1939.

74. Dunstan HP, Schneckloth RE, Corcoran AC, et al: The effectiveness of long-term treatment of malignant hypertension. Circulation 18:644–651, 1958.

75. Pierson EC, Hoobler SW: Significance of transient encephalopathy in cases of benign hypertension. Univ Michigan Med Bull 23:446–455, 1957.

76. Hoobler SW: Cooperative study on strokes and hypertension. Proceedings of Sixth Princeton Conference. In Cerebral Vascular Diseases, Toole JF, Siekert RG, Whisnant JP (eds), New York, Grune & Stratton, pp. 161–166, 1968.

77. Freis ED: Effect of treatment of hypertension on the occurrence of stroke. Proceedings of Ninth Princeton Conference. In Cerebral Vascular Diseases, Whisnant JP, Sandok BA (eds), New York, Grune & Stratton, pp. 133–136, 1974.

78. Marshall J: A trial of long-term hypotensive therapy in cerebrovascular disease. Lancet 1:10–12, 1964.

79. Hamilton M, Thompson EN, Wisnewski TKM: The role of blood pressure control in preventing complications of hypertension. Lancet 1:235–238, 1964.

80. Veterans Administration Cooperative Study Group on Antihypertensive Agents: Effects of treatment on morbidity in hypertension. I. Results in patients with diastolic blood pressures averaging 115 through 129 mm Hg. JAMA 202:1028–1034, 1967.

81. Veterans Administration Cooperative Study Group on Antihypertensive Agents: Results in patients with diastolic blood pressures averaging 90 through 114 mm Hg. JAMA 213:1143–1152, 1970.

82. The Management Committee: The Australian therapeutic trial in mild hypertension. Lancet 1:1261–1267, 1980.

83. Evans JG: Hypertension and stroke in an elderly population. Acta Med Scand (Suppl) 676:22–32, 1983.

84. Hodkinson HM, Exton-Smith AN: Factors predicting mortality in the elderly in the community. Age and Ageing 5:110–115, 1976.

85. Anderson F, Cowan NR: Survival of healthy older people. Brit J Prevent & Social Med 30:231–232, 1976.

86. Milne JS: A longitudinal study of blood pressure and stroke in older people. J Clin Experimental Gerontol 3:135–159, 1981.

8

Epidemiology of Stroke

As stated by Petlund:

Epidemiology contributes to the knowledge of a disease by

1—Demographic descriptions which give (a) an outline of the seriousness of the disease, and (b) guidance to health authorities

2—Giving cues to causal factors of the disease based on frequency and distribution.[1]

Accumulating data on large numbers of stroke patients has been a relatively recent occurrence and only a few such papers were published prior to the 1960s when articles from the Joint Study of Extracranial Arterial Occlusion began appearing in *JAMA* (see Chapter 4).

Newbill (1940) reviewed all cases of stroke in which autopsy studies were made at Charity Hospital between 1929 and 1938—a total of 296 cases.[2] He wanted to disprove the common belief that strokes are responsible for a great number of sudden deaths. Only one of these patients died in less than one hour after the onset of symptoms. This death occurred in 45 minutes and was the result of a hemorrhage in the pons of a black man, age 36, who, in addition, had syphilitic aortitis and arteriosclerotic heart disease. Newbill found that hemorrhage is more apt to be responsible if death occurs within 24 hours. The average survival after thrombosis is 15 times as long as after hemorrhage or embolism. There was a distinct difference in survival between males (57.3 days) and females (129.1 days).

Dalsgaard-Nielsen (1955) surveyed 1000 cases of stroke admitted to Frederiksberg Hospital during the period 1940 to 1953.[3] The material was catalogued by means of a punched-card system and over 200 items of information were included. The clinical criteria for the diagnosis (hemorrhage, thrombosis, embolism) are indicated. The data are discussed with reference to occupation, premorbid status, sex, age at onset of stroke, frequency of stroke, mortality, and poststroke status.

Although not published until 1971, Whisnant et al. reviewed records of the Mayo Clinic and other institutions in Olmsted County, Minnesota, for the years 1945 through 1954.[4] They identified 648 cases of stroke; in 98% medical care was received at Mayo Clinic at some time during the illness. There were 3 persons lost to follow-up, 184 alive in 1954, and 461 deceased. No significant differences were noted between men and women. Among those who survived the initial stroke, heart disease was the cause of nearly twice as many deaths as was subsequent stroke. From these and later studies, as well as from vital statistics, a wealth of information on stroke has been collected.

In the United States alone, approximately 400,000 new strokes occur each year and about 40% of those afflicted will die within 30 days. The age-adjusted death rates for cerebrovascular disease since 1900 are cited:[5,6]

Year	Per 100,000 population
1900	106.9
1920	93.0
1940	90.9
1960	79.7
1970	66.3
1982	35.8

Before 1940, the classification included "intracranial lesions of vascular origin." Since 1940, the category has been labeled "cerebrovascular diseases" and has included intracerebral and other intracranial hemorrhage, cerebral thrombosis and unspecified occlusion of cerebral arteries, and cerebral embolism.

As noted, death rates have been falling steadily in spite of the aging of the population. There is evidence for a decreasing incidence of both cerebral hemorrhage and cerebral thrombosis; this trend substantiates the declining death rates.[7] How long this decline has been in progress is anyone's guess, and this weakens all attempts to attribute the decrease to anything physicians or society have done. Subarachnoid hemorrhage, however, does not appear to share this downward course; its rates are either stable or possibly even increasing.[7]

Since hypertension is an important risk factor for stroke, the decline in mortality from stroke coupled with the emphasis on long-term treatment of hypertension has led to the assumption of a cause and effect relationship. A New Zealand study suggests that less than 10% of the observed decline in mortality from stroke between 1973 to 1982 in persons aged 30 to 60 resulted from an increase in the proportion of people receiving pharmacologic treatment for hypertension.[8] Miller and Kuller (1973) state:

> Since stroke deaths began to decline before the introduction of effective antihypertensive medication on a large scale and the rate of decline has not changed appreciably since the introduction of such drugs, improved treatment of hypertensive disease is not the major reason for the decrease in stroke rates.[9]

Data indicate also that in the United States hypertension has been declining for many years. The decline is apparent in both sexes and in both whites and nonwhites at all ages. The administration of antihypertensive therapy fails to explain the consistent downward slope in hypertensive deaths dating back at least to 1950 and probably several decades before that. The decrease in hypertension certainly affects the decline in atherothrombotic disease, but hypertension was declining while atherothrombosis was still rising.[10]

Most of us are willing to accept that diphtheria mortality rose to a peak in 1870 and has fallen quite regularly ever since, leaving us with no sufficient explanation for its coming and going. Perhaps, we will be obliged to accept that in a similar manner mysterious powers govern the ebb and flow of some noninfectious diseases.[10] Certainly, the diagnosis of acute myocardial infarction came on the scene around 1915 and rose over several decades but now has been declining for the past 15 to 20 years.

Data on the incidence of stroke worldwide are relatively abundant, but their comparability is rather poor because of the different diagnostic criteria, the age–sex breakdown, and the manner of reporting.[11] In many countries, a marked decrease in death rates has been shown during the last 30 years, but in others, mainly developing countries, they are still rising. In general, the highest incidence rates are those observed in Japanese and Chinese population cohorts.

Worldwide stroke mortality rates are about 100 deaths/100,000 population/year.[12] Fratiglioni et al. (1983) calculated average annual cerebrovascular disease mortality rates (age-adjusted to 1950 U.S. population) using data from 1967 to 1973 for 33 countries.[13] Rates ranged from 35.8/100,000/year (Philippines) to 196.7/100,000/year (Japan). Most of the age-adjusted incidence rates approximate 200 cases/100,000/year.[14]

A door-to-door survey was carried out in six cities of the People's Republic of China under the auspices of the World Health Organization.

There was 100% cooperation. The highest point prevalence ratio and incidence rate (age-adjusted to the 1960 U.S. population) was documented in the city of Harbin (441/100,000/year). While new strokes were primarily cerebral infarctions, the percentage of intracerebral hemorrhage (44%) was much greater than that reported among Caucasian populations.[15]

It is probable that the case-searching methods in China, and perhaps Japan, were more thorough than those of other countries. In some countries, hospitalized patients serve as the source of cases. Patients with mild strokes may not be hospitalized, and some persons with fatal strokes may die before reaching a hospital. Therefore, the high incidence reports from China and Japan may simply be more complete than those of the United States and Europe. Worldwide comparisons are flawed by this lack of uniformity in reporting of cases and also by the variation in the diagnostic criteria for stroke.[16]

Age-specific mortality rates reveal an exponentially increasing rate with increasing age.[12] For every five-year increase in age, the death rate for cerebrovascular disease approximately doubles.[12,17,18]

Schoenberg (1979) states that death data analyzed by sex reveal a slight excess in mortality for cerebrovascular disease among males. He believes that this slight difference is remarkable when contrasted to the conspicuous differential by sex (with a large male predominance) in mortality for cardiovascular disease and writes, "The reason for the large discrepancy in the sex distribution between cerebrovascular disease and cardiovascular disease remains unknown."[12] However, Alter et al. (1986) report that in 37 regions of the world reviewed by them, in all but one area, the standardized incidence ratios of stroke for men were greater than those for women.[16] The apparent male excess in stroke was significant by the Spearman rank order correlation test ($p = 0.001$). The incidence of initial stroke, which is about 40% higher for men than for women, was much greater for men in Japan (70%).

In analyzing U.S. mortality data by race, blacks generally have higher death rates than whites of the same age and sex and living in the same geographic region.[9,12] Southeastern areas of the United States have higher rates than other regions. Although this finding was initially thought to represent differences in death certificate practices, subsequent studies have revealed that this is not the case.[12,19]

Many physicians believe that stroke is a major problem of technically developed countries and that it is nonexistent or rare in Africa. A World Health Organization cooperative study of stroke registration in 14 centers worldwide showed that stroke in Nigeria equals the figures in European countries.[20] Data from centers in Mongolia, India, and Sri Lanka show that stroke is an important health problem in populations where athero-sclerosis is uncommon. However, hypertension is a global phenomenon, occurring at similar rates in probably most populations of the world. This study also revealed that the incidence of stroke in Japan has been over-estimated.

The cerebrovascular mortality rate of Japanese who migrate to Hawaii or California is substantially lower than that of their counterparts who remain behind.[12,21] However, the Japanese residing in California have higher blood pressures and blood cholesterol levels than those living in Hawaii or Japan.[22,23] The stroke mortality rates are perplexing and statistics such as these lead investigators to surmise that, perhaps, unknown risk factors are involved.[12]

According to Stallones (Figure 8.1):

A consistent finding of epidemiological studies of stroke is a strong relation with cardiac disease. Heart disease can be viewed as a characteristic that increases the risk of stroke, but a more appealing concept is that the dis-

Figure 8.1. REUEL A. STALLONES
(Courtesy of The University of Texas School of Public Health)

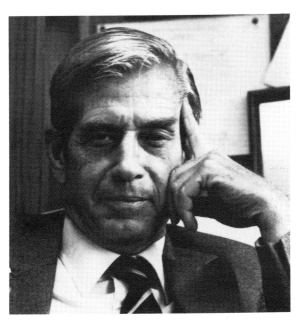

eases are linked through common precursors, e.g., hypertension and the correlates of occlusive arterial disease. Indeed these linkages are so strong that differences in the epidemiological features of stroke and cardio-vascular disease are more surprising than the similarities.

> Stroke may be examined as a part of a complex of vascular diseases rather than as a separate entity.[10]

Adams and associates (1984) state, "Because the long-term primary cause of death [in patients with TIAs] is myocardial infarction, it is likely that the most important way to prolong survival may be the vigorous investigation of their cardiac status and the treatment of their coronary artery disease even if asymptomatic."[24] Rolak et al. (1983) performed exercise-thallium-201 scintiscans and exercise-equilibrium radionuclide ventriculograms in 47 patients with TIAs or mild strokes.[25] Thirteen of 15 persons who had clinical evidence of heart disease and 14 of 32 persons without symptoms of coronary artery disease had abnormal studies. Coronary arteriography confirmed high-grade stenotic lesions (>70% stenosis) in 17 of 20 patients studied. In all, 57% of patients with TIAs or minor strokes had significant coronary artery disease.

In the management of stroke, no approach is as important as prevention. Treating risk factors that are believed to be forerunners of stroke is infinitely preferable to dealing with the consequences of a damaged brain. The Framingham study suggests that 10% of the asymptomatic population in which 50% of all strokes will occur can be identified.[26] Communities should be screened to find these individuals, and they (along with persons who are symptomatic from stroke risk factors) should have vigilant therapy. Programs of screening and prophylaxis would undoubtedly be less expensive than dealing with the acute care and long-term disability of stroke victims. When medical expenses are combined with lost income and productivity, the total cost of stroke in the United States, for example, is estimated to be $14 billion a year.[27] No one, however, can really calculate the cost to patients and families in terms of suffering, lost careers, and altered lives.

References

1. Petlund CF: Epidemiologic investigation of stroke. Scand J Rehabil Med (Suppl) 7:11–14, 1980.

2. Newbill HP: The duration of life after cerebrovascular accidents. JAMA 114:236–237, 1940.

3. Dalsgaard-Nielsen T: Survey of 1000 cases of apoplexia cerebri. Acta Psychiat et Neurol 30:169–185, 1955.

4. Whisnant JP, Fitzgibbons JP, Kurland LT, et al: Natural history of stroke in Rochester, Minnesota, 1945 through 1954. Stroke 2:11–22, 1971.

5. U.S. Department of Commerce, Bureau of Census: Vital Statistic Rates in the United States 1900–1940.

6. U.S. Department of Commerce, Bureau of Census: Statistical Abstract of the United States, p. 73, 1986.

7. Kurtzke JF: Epidemiology of Cerebrovascular Disease. Cerebrovascular Survey Report for Joint Council Subcommittee on Cerebrovascular Disease. National Institute of Neurological and Communicative Disorders and Stroke and National Heart and Lung Institute, pp. 135–176, January 1980.

8. Bonita R, Beaglehole R: Does treatment of hypertension explain the decline in mortality from stroke? Brit Med J 292:191–192, 1986.

9. Miller GD, Kuller LH: Trends in mortality from stroke in Baltimore, Maryland: 1940–1941 through 1968–1969. Am J Epidemiol 98:233–242, 1973.

10. Stallones RA: Epidemiology of stroke in relation to the cardiovascular disease complex. Adv Neurol 25:117–126, 1979.

11. Menotti A, Giampaoli S: Epidemiology and prediction of cerebral and peripheral vascular diseases. Monogr Atheroscler 14:11–14, 1986.

12. Schoenberg BS: Epidemiology of cerebrovascular disease. South Med J 72:331–336, 1979.

13. Fratiglioni L, Massey EW, Schoenberg DG, et al: Mortality from cerebrovascular disease; international comparisons and temporal trends. Neuroepidem 2:101–116, 1983.

14. Kurtzke JF: An introduction to the epidemiology of cerebrovascular disease. Proceedings of Tenth Princeton Conference. In Cerebral Vascular Diseases, Scheinberg P (ed), New York, Raven Press, pp. 239–253, 1976.

15. Li SC, Schoenberg BS, Wang CC, et al: Cerebrovascular disease in the People's Republic of China: Epidemiologic and clinical features. Neurology 35:1708–1713, 1985.

16. Alter M, Zhang ZX, Sobel E, et al: Standardized incidence ratios of stroke: A worldwide review. Neuroepidem 5:148–158, 1986.

17. Kurtzke JF: Epidemiology of Cerebrovascular Disease. Berlin, Springer-Verlag, 1969.

18. Petlund CF: Prevalence and Invalidity from Stroke in Aust-Adger County of Norway. Oslo, Universitetsforlaget, 1970.

19. Acheson RM, Nefzger MD, Heyman A: Mortality from stroke among U.S. veterans in Georgia and 5 western states. J Chronic Dis 26:405–414, 1973.

20. Lambo TA: Stroke—a worldwide health problem. Adv Neurol 25:1–3, 1979.

21. Worth RM, Kato H, Rhoads GG, et al: Epidemiologic studies of coronary heart disease and stroke in Japanese men living in Japan, Hawaii, and California: Mortality. Am J Epidemiol 102:481–490, 1975.

22. Marmot MG, Syme SL, Kagan A, et al: Epidemiologic studies of coronary heart disease and stroke in Japanese men living in Japan, Hawaii, and California: Prevalence of coronary and hypertensive heart disease and associated risk factors. Am J Epidemiol 102:514–525, 1975.

23. Nichaman MZ, Hamilton HB, Kagan A, et al: Epidemiologic studies of coronary heart disease and stroke in Japanese men living in Japan, Hawaii, and California: Distribution of biochemical risk factors. Am J Epidemiol 102:491–501, 1975.

24. Adams HP Jr, Kassell NF, Mazuz H: The patient with transient ischemic attacks—Is this the time for a new therapeutic approach? Stroke 15:371–375, 1984.

25. Rolak L, Rokey R, Verani M, et al: Coronary artery disease in patients with cerebrovascular disease. A prospective study. Ann Neurol 14:132, 1983 (abstract).

26. Wolf PA, Dawber TR, Kannel WB, et al: Epidemiologic assessment of the stroke candidate. Neurology 23:418, 1973 (abstract).

27. Office of Scientific and Health Reports, National Institute of Neurological and Communicative Disorders and Stroke: Stroke: Hope through research. NIH publication No. 83–2222, August 1983.

9

Well-Known Persons Who Have Suffered Strokes

Strokes have frequently been mentioned in descriptions of the illnesses and deaths of renowned persons. Some of the most interesting accounts are included in this chapter.

Marcello Malpighi

The greatest of the early microscopists, Malpighi discovered the capillaries and described the minute structure of the lungs, kidney, and spleen (Figure 9.1). This report of the strokes experienced by Malpighi, and of the postmortem findings, was written by Johann Jacob Wepfer in 1694 and translated into English in 1704.[1] This composition is taken from *Classic Descriptions of Disease* by R. H. Major.

> Marcellus Malpighi was of a Constitution that tended to a Dryness, an indifferent Habit of Body and a middling Stature; He had been subject for many Years to Vomiting, bilious Stools, Palpitations of the Heart, Stones in the Kidneys and Bladder, a pissing of Blood, and some light Touches of the Gout. Upon his coming to Rome, all these Disorders were inflam'd; especially the Palpitations of the Heart, the Stone in the Kidneys, and with sharp biting Night Sweats. Such was the Condition of Malpighi, July 25th, 1694, at which Time he was seiz'd, in the 66th Year of his Age, about 1 a Clock in the Afternoon, with an Apoplexy, usher'd in with Care, Passions of the mind, etc. The Apoplexy was attended with a Palsie of the whole right Side, and a Distortion of the Mouth and right Eye. Presently we try'd several Remedies, particularly Bleeding in the left Arm: If it had not been for the contrary Sentiments of the Physicians that consulted with

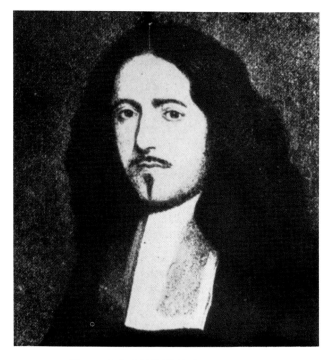

Figure 9.1. MARCELLO MALPIGHI
(From Clendening L: *Behind the Doctor*, 1933. Courtesy of Alfred A. Knopf, Publisher, New York)

me, I would have ordered the Blood to be drawn from the paralytick Arm; upon the Consideration, that the defective Circulation of the Fluids of the Part affected, is not retriev'd by any speedier Method than that of opening a Vein in the same; as it appears plainly from the mechanical Principles of Resistance and Motion. We prescrib'd at the same time scarrify'd Cupping-Glasies, to be applied to the Shoulder-Blades; the Powder of *Cornachini, Sinapismus's* to be apply'd to the Soles of the Feet; and several other spirituous, cephalick, and specifick Remedies; by the Use of which, after struggling 40 Days with a long Train of grievous Symptoms, particularly a Light-Headedness, a *Capiplenium,* and other Accidents, he got clear of the Apoplexy, and Palsie, and the above-mention'd Symptoms. But as Evils use to spread and gain Ground, so this famous Man suffer'd much by the fore-going Disease in his Memory and Reason, and melted into Tears upon the slightest Occasion. He was troubled by Intervals with Inappetency, a Want of Digestion in the Ventricle, a subsultory Motion of the Muscles, and slight Fits of a Giddiness. In fine, being worn out with these and other Symptoms, he was seiz'd Nov. 29 with a fresh fit of an Apoplexy, after the Injection of a customary Glyster in the morning: This new fit was usher'd in by a grievous Vertigo, with a fit of the Stone in the Bladder for eight Days, and an Exasperation of the above-mention'd Symptoms. But the Apoplectick Fit was more dismal than all the other Symptoms, for in spite of all Remedies whatsoever, he dy'd four Hours after the Invasion.

THE DISSECTION OF THE CORPS

In Dissecting the Corps, I found the right part of the lungs somewhat slaggy and livid, especially the hinder part that adheres to the back. The Heart was larger than ordinary, especially the Walls of the left Ventricle, which were as thick as the Breadth of two Fingers. The Gall in the Gall-Bladder was very black: The left Kidney was in a natural State, but the right was half as big again as the left, and the Bason of it was so much dilated, that one might easily thrust 2 Fingers into it. Perhaps this Dilatation of the pelvis was the Occasion that as soon as the Stones were bred in the Kidneys, they presently slipt into the Bladder, and so sprung out from thence, which our excellent Friend had frequently own'd to me to be a Matter of Fact. In the Bladder we found a little Stone that had descended thither four Days before the Invasion of the last Apoplectick Fit, and by Descent exasperated his last Vertigoes. The rest of the natural Viscera were very well condition'd.

When I open'd his Head, I found, in the Cavity of the right Ventricle of the Brain, an Extravasation of about 2 pints of black clotted Blood, which was the Cause of his Apoplexy and his Death. In the left Ventricle we found about an Ounce and a half of yellowish Water, with a small Quantity of little Grains of Sand mix'd with it. The Blood Vessels of the Brain were dilated and broke on all Hands. The whole Compass of the *dura Mater* adhered, tenaciously and praeternaturally to the *Cranium*. And this is the Sum of what I observ'd in Dissecting his Corps, Dec. 7, 1694.[2]

Louis Pasteur

Pasteur (Figure 9.2) suffered his first stroke 27 years prior to his death, and some of his greatest contributions to science were achieved during the poststroke period. The following narrative was taken from facts presented in *Louis Pasteur: Founder of Bacteriology* by John Mann.[3]

At the age of 46 years, Pasteur had already discovered that "left-handed" crystals deviated light to the left and "right-handed" crystals deviated light to the right, he had investigated fermentation for the wine industry

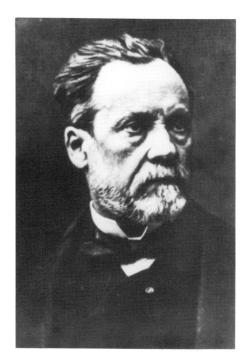

Figure 9.2. LOUIS PASTEUR
(From Cuny H: *Louis Pasteur: The Man and His Theories,* 1966. Courtesy of Les Éditions Robert Laffont, Paris)

and developed pasteurization, he had followed this inquiry further and had demonstrated the germ theory, and he was working on diseases of the silkworm.

Then, on October 19, 1868, Pasteur felt a strange tingling on his left side. He nevertheless wanted to go to the Academy of Sciences and read a paper by an Italian scientist who had used Pasteur's method of silkworm culture with great success. After his lunch, Pasteur had to lie down because he was shivering. Madame Pasteur was uneasy, and insisted that she walk with him to the Academy. There she asked a colleague to watch over her husband and see that he got home safely.

All the precautions seemed to have been unnecessary. Pasteur read the paper, returned home, had supper, and went to bed early. But as soon as he lay down, he found that he could not speak. His voice returned in a few minutes, and he called his wife. She hurriedly sent for a doctor.

Slowly Pasteur's entire left side became paralyzed. The diagnosis was that "he had had a cerebral hemorrhage; one of the blood vessels in his head was damaged and leaking blood." Other doctors were sent for.

Pasteur knew from the beginning both the nature of his affliction and the dimness of the hope for recovery, but his mind was not affected by the disaster overtaking his body. Three months later he was on his way back to the silkworm country. Pasteur had endured personal tragedy prior to his stroke, having lost his father and three young daughters. One child, Cécile, died of typhoid fever at the age of 13 years; Camille died in her second year of unknown cause; and Jeanne died at the age of nine years, but we were unable to find any reference to the cause of her death.

After recovery from his stroke, Pasteur completed and published his research on silkworm diseases and developed healthy moths to revitalize the industry for France and other countries; he developed chicken-cholera and anthrax vaccines and created the first vaccine for rabies.

On October 23, 1887, at the age of 65 years, Pasteur was suddenly struck dumb. He had just finished writing a letter. When he turned to say something to his wife, he discovered that he could not speak. He did not allow this attack, however, to keep him from an afternoon appointment with his daughter, since he did not want to frighten her. The day was spent quietly. Then, just as suddenly as it had left him, his speech returned toward evening. Two days later he was back at work with no signs of the episode, but a week later the paralysis recurred without warning.

Pasteur went on with his work, but at a slower pace. Daily, he walked to the Pasteur Institute to see patients receiving the rabies vaccine. He held the children's hands, dried their tears, and bid them a fond good-by when their cure was completed. On his seventieth birthday, a great celebration was held for him in the theater of the Sorbonne.

In 1895, he had an attack of uremia and, following this, he gradually grew weaker and slower. By the end of September, he was too weak to leave his bed. On September 27, when he was offered a cup of milk, he whispered, "I cannot." For a while he slept peacefully, but suddenly he began to gasp in agony and paralysis seized him. For 24 hours Pasteur lay motionless, his eyes closed. He died serenely the next day, September 28, 1895, and is buried in a marble crypt at the Pasteur Institute.

Vladimir Ilyich Lenin

In 1918, at the age of 48 years, Lenin survived an assassination attempt when a woman fired three shots from a revolver, one entering the left side of his neck, one lodging in his left shoulder, and the third passing through his coat.[4] His chauffeur drove him to the Kremlin and Lenin insisted on walking up two flights of stairs to his bedroom, with blood running down his shirt.[5] The bullets were left intact, and, after several months of convalescence, Lenin gradually resumed work.

In the winter of 1921 Lenin began suffering from insomnia, nausea, fainting spells, and intense headaches; he was only 51.[6] On May 26, 1922, a physician visited Lenin because of abdominal pain and vomiting. On examination, the doctor noted some slurring of speech and a mild right hemiparesis—his first stroke. Prolonged rest was advised, but, in the fall, he was allowed to return to work on a reduced schedule.

In the latter part of November it was noted that "often as he spoke the words were slurred, and he paused several times like a man who has lost the thread of his argument. He looked gaunt and frail."[5] He was ordered to bed with absolutely no work. On December 13 he had two attacks of nausea and vomiting; insomnia and headaches had returned. On December 16, 1922, there were visible signs of paralysis on the right side; the slight weakness became a definite hemiplegia—his second stroke.

Lenin had gradually come to realize that he had committed a grave error in assigning a high position to Stalin. After his second stroke he feared that the succession would go to Stalin and he abhorred the idea of surrendering Russia to a man who was so coarse, so uncultured, and so unprincipled. The word he used to describe Stalin was "grub," which is more than "rude." Lenin wrote:

> Stalin is too coarse, and this fault, though tolerable in dealings among us Communists, becomes unbearable in a General Secretary. Therefore, I propose to the comrades to find some way of removing Stalin from his position and appointing somebody else who differs in all respects from Comrade Stalin in one characteristic—namely, someone more tolerant, more loyal, more polite and considerate to his comrades, less capricious, etc.[5]

Following his second stroke, physicians insisted on absolute rest for Lenin. He was isolated in his home at Gorki and was to receive neither visitors nor political information (Figure 9.3). However, he continued dictating notes for a few minutes each day and some of these contained references against Stalin.

On March 9, 1923, Lenin suffered his third stroke, which deprived him of the power of speech, completely paralyzed his right side, and partially affected his left side.[5] For two months he was dreadfully ill but slowly some strength returned, and by the end of July he could walk a little. In the beginning of October he seemed to be recovering well. There was no

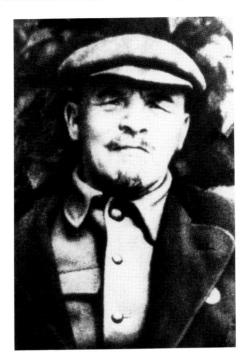

Figure 9.3. VLADIMIR ILYICH LENIN AT GORKI, AUGUST 1922
(From *The Life and Death of Lenin,* R. Payne, 1964, with permission of Ernst,
Cane, Gitlin, and Winick, New York)

paralysis on his left side and he walked easily with a cane. He understood
perfectly what people were saying but was able to enunciate only a few
simple words. (One of the authors, W. S. Fields, visited the home at
Gorki in 1972 and was surprised to see a direct telephone line to the
Kremlin; this had been installed after his third stroke in the event that his
speech might be restored.) Lenin had so improved that on October 19 he
was driven to Moscow to visit an agricultural exhibition and then for a
brief stop at the Kremlin.[5]

As Lenin improved, Stalin's concern must have increased. It would be
of inestimable value to Stalin if Lenin should die, and from this has come
considerable speculation as to whether Lenin's sudden demise in January
1924 was not at the instigation of Stalin.[6]

On January 21, 1924, Lenin had only a few sips of tea in the morning
and a few morsels of food for lunch; he was in bed most of the day,

sleeping or dozing. Around 6:00 P.M. the servants noticed some difficulty breathing and a physician was summoned. Soon, breathing became labored and then frantic; he was unresponsive and convulsions occurred. He died at 6:50 P.M.

The circumstances and rapidity of his death aroused suspicion that Stalin may have been responsible and poisoning has been seriously considered. Death occurred at a time when Trotsky (a close friend of Lenin) was absent from Moscow, and the Soviet secret police agent, assigned to guard Lenin, was a former pharmacist capable of mixing a poison.[4]

The necropsy report referred to generalized arteriosclerosis, multiple foci of yellow cerebromalacia of the left cerebral hemisphere, a fresh hemorrhage into the vascular plexus overlying the corpora quadrigemina, and stated that "the left internal carotid artery in its intracranial course has a completely obliterated lumen."[5] Lenin was a relatively young victim of atherosclerosis, and several details are curious. A prominent ophthalmologist had followed Lenin for some years and, in fact, saw him the day before his death. The professor "maintained that till the very end there were no visible pathological changes in Lenin's eyes."[7] Also, in 1922, before the first stroke, a shrewd physician (Professor Felix Klemperer) had apparently ignored the diagnosis of arteriosclerosis and expressed a belief that the bullets which had been lodged in Lenin since 1918 were poisoned. The bullet above the right clavicle was accordingly removed.[4] We may dismiss this suggestion as ridiculous, but as stated by L'Etang, "One cannot ignore the clinical judgment of an experienced observer."[4] Klemperer may have been instinctively correct in relating the bullets to Lenin's illness though incorrect about the poisoning. The track of one bullet has been recorded:

> One bullet had passed through his neck from left to right, missing the aorta by a fraction of an inch, and after piercing the lung it lodged in the neck, above the right clavicle.[5]

It is not inconceivable that the left internal carotid artery may have been damaged by the bullet, leading to a gradually increasing and spreading thrombosis in an arterial tree that already bore the changes of atherosclerosis.[4] Some support for this theory was furnished by the Commissar of Health, who wrote in a popular article at the time that the internal carotid "had been blocked at the entrance to the brain."[7]

In a speech at Lenin's funeral, Stalin announced himself as commander of the faithful; it was many years before it became generally known that Lenin had vowed eternal enmity to Stalin.[5]

Josef Stalin

In spite of Lenin's contempt for this man, Stalin succeeded him as Secretary General of the Communist Party of the Union of Soviet Socialist Republics. Biographer Robert Payne describes Stalin:

> This small, brooding, pock-marked man with a crooked arm, black teeth and yellow eyes, was the greatest tyrant of his time, and perhaps of all time.[8]

Milovan Djilas, one of the leaders of the Yugoslav Communist Party and a close friend of Josip Broz Tito, wrote a book *Conversations with Stalin*.[9] Djilas subsequently had a change of heart about communism, fell out of favor with Tito, and was imprisoned for many years. Djilas wrote:

> . . . it was made public in Moscow that he [Stalin] had probably killed the Leningrad Secretary, Kirov, in order to gain a pretext for settling accounts with the intra-Party opposition. He probably had a hand in Gorky's death; that death was depicted too prominently in his propaganda as the work of the opposition. Trotsky even suspects that he killed Lenin, with the excuse that he was shortening his misery. It is claimed that he killed his own wife, or in any case, through his harshness, he caused her to kill herself.[9]

The following report of Stalin's medical history is taken primarily from biographies by Robert Payne,[8] Blaine Taylor,[10] and Adam B. Ulam.[11]

At the age of seven, Stalin had smallpox, which left disfiguring scars that were large and numerous; after he came to power, photographs had to be carefully retouched. Around the age of ten, an injury to his left arm was complicated by infection and blood poisoning. As a result, Josef's left arm was three inches shorter than the right, and he never had complete muscular control of his left hand; at times he wore a brace to support the elbow. It has been suggested by an orthopedic surgeon that Stalin suffered "a compound fracture with resultant osteomyelitis and a subsequent hand deformity secondary to disturbance of growth of the arm, the hand deformity being produced by a Volkmann's contracture subsequent to improper treatment of the fracture."[8] Stalin had been born into harsh, abject poverty, the son of a drunken father who beat him frequently, and one biographer believes the arm injury occurred during a ferocious beating by his father.[8] At any rate, the arm was weak and caused him pain and discomfort throughout his life. The fact that he went to considerable trouble to attempt to hide his defect indicates that it probably had a profound effect on his emerging character.[8]

Josef Stalin's private life has been discussed in detail in his daughter's book (*20 Letters to a Friend*[12]) and in Khrushchev's memoirs (*Khrushchev Remembers*[13]). He ate huge meals with plenty of fruit and meat. He once dared Churchill to split a suckling pig with him, and, when Sir Winston refused, Stalin polished off the whole pig himself. He believed in drunkenness and claimed his father weaned him on vodka in his cradle. Khrushchev describes a late dinner, with Stalin becoming very drunk and the assembly ending at 5:00 or 6:00 A.M. (as was usual). He loved motion picture films, especially American westerns, and often watched two or three a night with his cronies in the Kremlin. Stalin was a bad husband; as a father, he was at times cruel, at other times doting. His hobbies were bowling, hunting, sitting in the garden, and walking in the woods.

On his seventy-third birthday on December 21, 1952, Josef Stalin "was one of the most powerful men on earth, the ruler of All the Russias whose armies occupied half of Europe and whose generals wanted him to take the rest of the world."[14] The first public indication of Stalin's failing health occurred when his daughter visited him around that time. Ulam records:

> She noticed changes. His usually gray, pale face was flushed. In retrospect, she believes it was a symptom of high blood pressure. But possibly it also reflected his internal agitation. He had stopped smoking, another sign that he felt his health to be failing.[11]

Bortoli gives us this sketch of the dictator in the last weeks of his life:

> In the morning, well rested, he still walked with a lively step. But, apart from that, he was an old man with a sallow, rough complextion [sic]. His hair was gray, but he did not bother to have it dyed. . . . Forced by the state of his health to stop smoking, he still flourished his pipe, which for so long a time had been an integral part of his personality and which he carried in his trouser pocket. He took care of himself in a rather anarchic fashion. For a while, he was interested in Bogomolet's studies on rejuvenation, and the laboratories of the Ukrainian professor were inundated with rubles. But, being suspicious, he put himself into doctors' hands as little as possible. Like many old people from that era, he thought he could treat his illnesses by swallowing a few drops of tincture of iodine in a glass of water.[15]

However, time was running out for Stalin. Author Hingley writes:

> The last independent witness—that is, the last person outside the Kremlin-instructed world—known to have set eyes on the living Stalin was the Indian Ambassador to Moscow whom the dictator received on February 17, 1953.[16]

Suddenly, without warning, Stalin dropped out of sight. The stroke that felled him occurred during the night of March 1, 1953. According to rumors, he remained unattended for many hours afterward because the guards, who became disturbed when he failed to ask for his late evening repast, did not dare to break open the locked ironplated door that led to his bedroom.[11] Stalin had been adamant in his orders that they should never awaken him. When security officers finally entered his room, Stalin was unconscious on the floor. It was mid-morning when his daughter and son were summoned.

Only when his condition was deemed hopeless, on March 4, did his colleagues communicate news of his illness to the world. On that day Tass, the official Soviet news agency, made a statement saying that:

> Comrade Stalin, while in his apartment in Moscow, was struck by a cerebral hemorrhage affecting the vital areas of his brain. Comrade Stalin has lost consciousness. His right arm and right leg have been paralyzed. He has lost the ability to speak. Serious cardiac and respiratory complications have arisen.[10]

Stalin died the next day, March 5, at 9:50 P.M.

Payne (cited by Taylor) writes that the autopsy report on Stalin is strikingly devoid of details:

> The description of the brain hemorrhage is so brief, and stated in such general terms, that it gives rise to the suspicion that the brain was not uncovered and examined, and the doctors merely contented themselves with opening up the body. . . . There may have been excellent reasons for not examining the brain. Stalin himself may have forbidden it in his testament knowing that Lenin's brain, cut into 30,000 slices, had become a plaything of the Brain Institute in Moscow. . . . The doctors may have been so awed in the presence of the dead Stalin that they could not and dared not open the skull case. It is possible that the complete autopsy was never published, and the published report merely indicates the doctors' conclusions. Finally, there is the possibility that the autopsy was fraudulent, and that Stalin did not die in the manner indicated. . . . Though we may never know exactly how Stalin died, or even the exact date of his death, there are indications that he died long before the evening of March 5, and it is possible that he died violently. . . .
>
> All the available evidence suggests that between February 25 and March 5 there was a vacuum of power. No one ruled, for no one dared to rule.[10]

Payne's conclusion is that the announcement of Stalin's incapacity and death was delayed for eight days, allowing the various Kremlin leadership factions to jockey for time, position, and power.[10]

Biographer Hingley seems to agree with Payne's overall conclusion on the timing of Stalin's death:

. . . suggests that Stalin suffered on or about 21 February some form of incapacitation which removed him from the control of events. Perhaps the stroke officially reported as occurring on the night of 1–2 March had in fact occurred a week earlier or perhaps there had been a previous, less severe, stroke.

It remains possible that [Laurenti] Beria or some other menaced individual found means to poison the dictator. No faith need be placed in the three official medical bulletins of 4–5 March. . . . Though the "best medical brains" were reported as attending the ailing dictator, it was far from clear why they described Stalin as having been robbed of consciousness before losing the power of speech; one does not need a medical degree to judge such a claim suspicious. And why, if Stalin indeed suffered the attack in his Moscow apartment, as reported in the first radio communiqué, was he removed to his Kuntsevo villa—from an area bristling with excellent facilities—which is where Svetlana Alliluyeva found her father dying?[16]

Further, Hingley reports that Stalin's alcoholic son "lurched around the bungalow, accusing his expiring father's entourage of murdering him by poison or other means."[16]

After all the speculation following Stalin's death, Taylor concludes:

What is certain, however, is that Stalin's death in 1953 helped reduce the then-growing risk of a new, more terrible world war, for as he told an intimate in 1944, referring to the still-raging World War II, "It'll take us 20 years to recover, then we'll have another go at it."
Consider the alternative: what might've happened if Stalin died at age 83, a decade later than he did?[10]

In more recent years, Stalin's body has been removed from the mausoleum where it rested next to Lenin's. Soviet leader Mikhail Gorbachev, like Nikita Khrushchev before him, has told the Soviet people that Josef Stalin committed "enormous and unforgivable" crimes; he announced that a top-level commission has been set up to investigate them.[17]

United States Presidents

The details of strokes suffered by presidents of the United States are noteworthy not only because of widespread interest in their lives but also because some of the strokes occurred during their terms of office and had serious influences on national and world concerns. We know of seven presidents and many first ladies who have had strokes. (Warren Harding is not included as the diagnosis in his case is questionable.) The following descriptions are taken primarily from the works of Dr. Rudolph Marx,[18] Dr. Charles W. Robertson,[19] and Dr. Morris Fishbein.[20]

John Quincy Adams

On November 20, 1846, at 79 years of age (17 years after leaving the White House), John Quincy Adams was visiting his son in Boston. He rose in the dark of the November morning, between four and five o'clock, bathed and rubbed himself vigorously with his horsehair mitten, and went down to breakfast. Later, out with a friend on a morning stroll, Adams suffered a stroke and fell down. He was taken to his son's house, where he remained in a coma for several days. He recovered slowly, and in about three months was again on his feet. In 1847, Adams returned to Washington and took up his post in Congress. He was the only president who, when his term ended, was not too proud to accept nomination to the House of Representatives, where he served for the remainder of his life. On February 21, 1848, the work of the House was interrupted by cries of "Stop! Look to Mr. Adams!" The old patriot, now 81 years old, had toppled over into the arms of a nearby member. A second stroke had felled him. He lived three days and was unconscious most of the time.

John Tyler

In 1820 (at the age of 30 years), while serving in Congress, John Tyler wrote to his family doctor back home in Virginia:

> I sustained a violent singular shock four days ago. I had gone to the House on Thursday morning having before experienced a disagreeable sensation in my head which increased so much as to force me to leave the hall. It then visited in succession the hands, feet, tongue and lips creating on each the effect which is produced by what is commonly called a "sleeping hand," which all of us are subject to. But it was so severe as to render my limbs, tongue, etc. almost useless to me. I was bled and took purgative medicines which have rendered me convalescent. The doctor here ascribed it to a diseased stomach and very probably correctly did so. I am now walking about and am to appearance well, but often experience a glow in my face and over the whole system which is often followed up by debility with pains in my neck and arms.[18]

In this instance, the diagnosis of food poisoning may have been correct. Certain toxins have a special affinity for the nervous system and may cause tingling and prickling sensations and numbness of the extremities, lips, and tongue. Another possibility is a stroke. Although Tyler was very young for this latter illness, he was slow in recuperating and felt weak and unwell for a long time thereafter.

Tyler became vice president in 1841, and then, upon William Henry Harrison's death from virus pneumonitis and hepatitis, he ascended to the presidency. When Tyler moved into the White House, his wife (mother of his seven children) was partially paralyzed from a stroke. After eighteen months of invalidism, another brain infarction ended her life. In 1844, the 54-year-old president married a 24-year-old woman who also bore him seven children.

In January 1862 (17 years after leaving the presidency), while staying at the Exchange Hotel in Richmond, Tyler experienced an episode during which he felt dizzy and nauseated and vomited bile. Having had similar dizzy spells, he made light of it and went downstairs to the dining room for a cup of tea. While drinking it, he suddenly lost consciousness and slumped to the floor. After a few moments he opened his eyes and insisted on climbing the stairs to his room. Four physicians examined him and made a diagnosis of biliousness. The patient was permitted to be up and around, but after a few days he was put to bed because he complained about headaches and cough. On January 17, 1862, he was aroused from sleep by a feeling of suffocation and breathing ceased.

In retrospect, it was believed that Tyler's previous dizzy spells may have been TIAs, and that, in the dining room, he had had a major stroke affecting the frontal lobe. The final event may have been an extension of a vascular thrombosis paralyzing the respiratory center.

Millard Fillmore

This president was a health addict who did not smoke or drink but preferred milk and simple foods. Although overweight, he enjoyed good health up to his last sickness. Twenty years after his presidential term, on the morning of February 13, 1874, after Fillmore had finished shaving, his left hand suddenly dropped powerless to his side. The paralysis soon spread to the left side of his face and to the muscles of the larynx and pharynx, making breathing and swallowing difficult. The symptoms indicated involvement of centers in the medulla. There was temporary improvement, then the patient sustained another stroke two weeks later that resulted in paralysis of the entire left side of his body. He was unconscious for 24 hours and thereafter was unable to leave his bed. Fillmore died on March 8, 1874, at the age of 74.

Andrew Johnson

History has recorded that Andrew Johnson was under the influence of alcohol when he gave his rambling inauguration speech as vice president. However, his doctor apparently had advised him to take a tumblerful of whiskey that morning because he felt faint with diarrhea and cramps. He had been suffering from a chronic gastrointestinal infection during the previous five months and arrived at Washington sick and weary. Unfortunately, Johnson's political foes didn't miss the chance to keep reiterating that he made a fool of himself at his inauguration and had disgraced the dignity of his office. The American people perceived him forever as a drunkard. He suffered much harassment while in office and endured the humiliation of a Senate impeachment trial, which he won by a single vote.

After leaving the White House in 1869, Johnson returned to Tennessee and in 1874, at age 66, won election to the Senate; he was the only former president to achieve this distinction.

On July 30, 1875, while visiting his daughter, he went to his room to rest after lunch. His granddaughter talked with him as he sat in an armchair. As she turned to leave the room, he fell forward on the carpet and was lying helpless, his left side paralyzed. He remained conscious and able to speak and sternly forbade the family to get a physician. The next day a second stroke paralyzed his whole body and blacked out his consciousness. Physicians were summoned, and he was treated by bleeding. In two hours he was dead.

Chester Alan Arthur

In 1881, following the assassination of James Garfield, Arthur assumed the presidency. He loved heavy foods, fine wines and after-dinner liqueurs, disregarding his expanding girth. Inevitably, overweight, overwork, and too many parties took their toll. In 1883, the 53-year-old president was worn out, and his doctors sent him to Florida to recuperate. During his vacation he contracted a severe type of malaria unresponsive to quinine. He returned home a very sick man and recovered at a slow pace.

Subsequently, he suffered from frequent attacks of epigastric pain, diagnosed by his doctors as nervous indigestion, but which may have been chronic gallbladder disease. When he was not nominated for a second term, Arthur returned to his law practice in New York, retiring after a few months because of ill health.

At age 55 he developed acute nephritis and, subsequently, congestive heart failure. Arthur was in constant misery, and in June 1886 said despondently to a friend, "After all, life is not worth living. I might as well give up the struggle for it now as at any other time and submit to the inevitable."[18] On November 16, 1886, while sleeping, he suffered a hemorrhagic stroke that paralyzed his left side and rendered him unconscious. He died two days later.

Woodrow Wilson

This account has been excerpted from Gene Smith's interesting book, *When the Cheering Stopped: The Last Years of Woodrow Wilson.*[21]

Wilson died in 1924 at the age of 67. He suffered a stroke in September 1919, while on an exhausting whistle-stop tour of the country. He was attempting to rally the electorate to support his efforts to put the United States into the League of Nations over the objections of many senators. Wilson (Figure 9.4) had spent the first six months of 1919 in Europe participating in interminable talks, meetings, and arguments with officials of several countries trying to negotiate territorial claims at the close of World War I. Under unrelenting stress, a muscle twitching around his left eye spread to become a spasmodic jerking of half of his face; he complained constantly of severe headache. (The muscle twitching had been present since 1906 when an ophthalmic artery thrombosis resulted in blindness of that eye.)

On September 25, 1919, in Pueblo, Colorado, he stumbled slightly at the single step leading into the Memorial Auditorium. A Secret Service agent caught him and almost lifted him up over the step. His address to the large audience went smoothly until he suddenly faltered:

> Germany must never be allowed—(He stopped and was silent.) A lesson must be taught to Germany—(He stopped again and stood still.) The world will never allow Germany—(This had never happened before in any of his speeches. The President gathered himself together and went on. When he finished his speech, the President was crying.)[21]

That night he called to his wife, "Can you come to me, Edith? I'm terribly sick." He was sitting on the edge of his bed with his head resting on the back of a chair. He had a "splitting agony" in his head. Mrs. Wilson and his physician tried to ease his discomfort by propping him

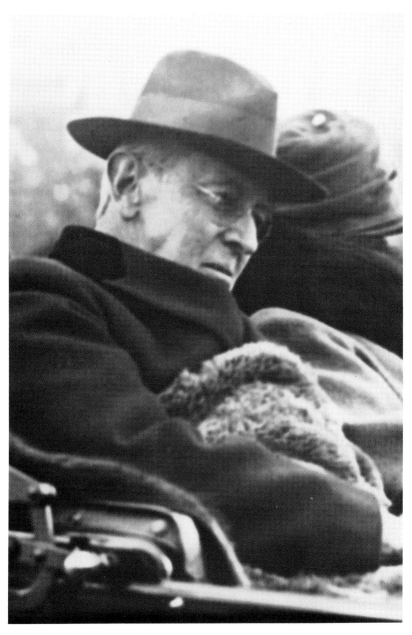

Figure 9.4. WOODROW WILSON
(With permission of the Woodrow Wilson Collection of the Library of Congress)

up with a pillow, and about 5:00 A.M. he finally fell asleep. When the room grew light, he managed to get up and shave, but when he returned from the bathroom "saliva came down from the left side of his mouth and the left half of his face was fallen and unmoving. His words were mumbled and indistinct."[21] His left arm and leg hung useless.

His physician said, "The President has suffered a complete nervous breakdown."[21] The remainder of the tour was cancelled, and the train returned to Washington, a two-day journey. During this period, some function returned to his arm and leg, and he was able to walk with his daughter to an open car at Washington's Union Station. It was Sunday morning and the streets were almost empty, but as they rode to the White House, the president "took off his hat and bowed as if he were returning the greetings of a vast throng. Enough people saw what he had done to send flying through Washington the information that the President is physically all right but salutes empty sidewalks. He has lost his mind."[21]

The next few days he did little official work; he could use his left arm and leg but still complained of the pain in his head and spent most of the time in his room and study. When he awoke on October 2, his left hand hung loosely and he told his wife that he had no feeling in it. He went into the bathroom and the doctor was summoned. Before the physician arrived, Mrs. Wilson heard a noise in the bathroom, rushed in and found the president lying unconscious on the floor. The first lady and an aide lifted President Wilson to his bed. When the physician arrived, he gasped, "My God, the President is paralyzed."[21]

Other physicians were called in for consultation, but they released no information and nothing could be ascertained beyond the fact that the president was ill. Daily bulletins were posted giving noncommittal statements that the president had a fairly good night or that he had remained in bed all day. The Secretary of State, Robert Lansing, called a cabinet meeting to discuss the question of President Wilson's ability to discharge his duties. The cabinet made repeated requests for detailed information about his diagnosis but had no success. The official physician said that the president was suffering from a nervous breakdown, indigestion, and a depleted system; that it was "touch and go," the "scales might tip either way and they might tip the wrong way" if the president was harassed by business matters.

The press, congressmen, and cabinet members complained about the vague generalities but were not enlightened further. Vice President Thomas R. Marshall was a former governor of Indiana and was accustomed to spending little time in Washington. He had attended a few cabinet meetings when President Wilson was in Europe for the Peace Conference but was upset at the thought of assuming the role of chief executive. Marshall stated that he would take over only if there was a congressional resolution approved in writing by President Wilson's physician and Mrs. Wilson.

The president's doctor was a naval officer on active duty, sworn to obey the orders of his commander in chief and, therefore, voiceless in policy matters. He stated that he would never certify to the patient's disability. The president himself was desperately ill and unable to decide anything. There was only one person who could speak in his name and use his powers as president; only one person who could decide that he would continue in his job as though nothing had happened. His wife (Edith Galt Wilson) made this decision. She guarded the door to his room and gave no access to his secretary or any government officials. Documents and urgent letters were sent to his room, but most were ignored; decision making was put off and put off.

By the end of October 1919, Wilson could sign his name with the first lady steadying his right hand. On October 30 he received the King and Queen of Belgium and on November 13, the Prince of Wales. Members of the cabinet were not permitted to see him but were received by Mrs. Wilson, who relayed messages back and forth.

In February 1921, the president, for the first time in 17 months, walked to the executive wing of the White House for a cabinet meeting, a walk of 600 yards. He moved slowly with little assistance, the left foot dragging. One by one he invited the men to lunch. March 3 was his last full day as president. He was succeeded by Warren G. Harding.

On February 3, 1924, Woodrow Wilson died from a massive infarction of the brain. In retrospect, it was believed that Wilson had suffered his first stroke in April 1919 while in Paris at the Peace Conference. His illness at that time was diagnosed as influenza, but after the acute sickness peculiar actions were noted—he thought furniture was being stolen from the house he occupied; he became obsessed with the idea that the French servants were all spies; he insisted that official cars not be used for formerly permitted pleasure trips; and he banished a close friend (Colonel Edward House) from his confidence. He became very irritable and suspicious.

After his major stroke in September 1919, Wilson became more unreasonable and emotional, with frequent crying spells; he lost a great deal of his judgmental and evaluating skill, but never lost his delightful sense of humor. Throughout the period subsequent to this stroke, he was in no condition to fulfill the obligations of the presidency.

Warren G. Harding

Opinions differ on the immediate cause of President Harding's sudden death in 1923. It is said that a famous heart specialist, Dr. Emmanuel Libmann of New York, met Harding at a dinner party in the fall of 1922 and expressed his private judgment that the president had severe coronary artery disease and would be dead in six months. The chief executive did succumb in eight months.

Harding was a playboy at heart, fond of liquor, rich food, and poker parties with his cronies. His weakness of character, which resulted in several sordid situations in his private life, also bred an epidemic of scandals and corruption during his administration.

We do not know when he first began to have symptoms of heart disease. In January 1922 he had a serious illness; it was diagnosed as influenza accompanied by digestive disorders and kidney complications. Thereafter, he became increasingly listless and easily exhausted. Physical effort and emotional stress sometimes caused short periods of pain in the middle of his chest, which made him stop in his tracks and remain quiet until the pain vanished. The president's physician, Surgeon General Charles E. Sawyer, must have recognized these episodes as typical of angina pectoris; he knew also that Harding's systolic blood pressure had been around 180 mm Hg for some years. The president had shortness of breath on slight exertion, and for several months before his death had propped himself up with several pillows in order to sleep.[18]

In July 1923, Harding took a trip by train and boat to Alaska and then back to Seattle. On the morning of July 28, he was suddenly awakened by an attack of pain in the lower chest and upper abdomen. It started like his previous seizures of angina but continued and increased in severity. He became deathly pale with a bluish hue and broke out in cold perspiration. Nausea and vomiting ensued and these gastric symptoms convinced Dr. Sawyer that this was an attack of acute indigestion.

In the president's party, however, a young physician, Commander Joel T. Boone, found the president's heart sounds feeble and blood pressure at shock level. He diagnosed the episode as cardiac and confidentially advised others of the gravity of the situation. Apparently, Dr. Sawyer permitted the patient to get up; no strict bed rest was enforced during the first three days.

Harding was put to bed on a special train for the trip back to Washington, but at a stopover in San Francisco was permitted to walk from the train to a car and also from the automobile to the elevator and to his room in the Palace Hotel. This physical effort may have aggravated his condition, for the chest pain returned; fever, bronchopneumonia, Cheyne-Stokes respiration, heart failure, and pulmonary edema developed. At last, bed rest was mandated and heart stimulants were injected. He improved rapidly and by the sixth day of his illness was comfortable and asymptomatic. Suddenly, that evening, a convulsive tremor passed over Harding's face; his body shuddered and sagged. He was dead at age 58.

Mrs. Harding would not permit an autopsy. The official statement of his physicians said, "We all believe he died from apoplexy or the rupture of a blood vessel in the axis of the brain near the respiratory center."[19] Although the electrocardiograph had been demonstrated in the United States in 1918, no electrocardiogram was taken of the stricken President Harding during the six days of his illness in 1923.

Dr. Rudolph Marx believes that his sudden demise was caused by a complication of the unrecognized coronary thrombosis:

> The occurrence of a catastrophe on the sixth day of a patient who was permitted to walk around during the first three days, and suffering from high blood pressure, suggests a massive rupture of a softened infarct in the wall of the heart. It is noteworthy that one of his sisters died suddenly and unexpectedly in the same way.[18]

Franklin Delano Roosevelt

It appears that from birth Roosevelt had a chronic weakness of his respiratory tract, and historical accounts of his childhood as well as his personal letters during adult life are filled with complaints of colds, sore throats, sinus trouble, bronchitis, and fever. At age 39 he was stricken with paralytic poliomyelitis and was never again able to walk without assistance. He showed great courage, and it appears that his illness taught him to laugh at all obstacles and never to accept defeat. He reportedly said, "If you had spent two years in bed trying to wiggle your big toe, after that everything else would seem easy."[18]

An assassination attempt on Roosevelt's life took place in Miami, Florida, in February 1932, a few weeks before his inauguration. He had just given a short talk from the rear seat of his automobile when five bullets from the assassin's revolver mortally wounded Mayor Anton Cermak of Chicago and injured four bystanders. Immediately, the FBI wanted to rush Roosevelt out of harm's way, but he insisted on getting his bleeding friend Cermak to the hospital in the car, holding him in his strong arms all the way.

During his twelve years in the White House FDR was under the constant care of the Surgeon General of the Navy, Dr. Ross T. McIntyre, an eye, nose, and throat specialist. In 1937 it was reported that the president's blood pressure had shown a slight rise; simultaneously he gained weight and had to start dieting. It is said that in 1938, while visiting his son at the Mayo Clinic, the first of a series of "little strokes" occurred.

It was midway through the war, in 1943, that a definite physical change in Roosevelt's appearance was obvious, particularly following a trip to Cairo and Teheran. Dr. Charles W. Robertson states, "It seems quite plain that Roosevelt suffered a series of small strokes in 1943 and 1944."[19] In December 1943 he had an influenza-like attack of two weeks' duration and lost about ten pounds. Several doctors were called in for consultation. All refused to disclose information for publication but intimated that the president had symptoms of cerebral arteriosclerosis with vascular cerebral insufficiency.

In the spring of 1944 the chief executive developed a severe bronchitis that gave the appearance of bronchopneumonia. He was seriously ill. He recovered slowly and incompletely, and his cough persisted. In the fall of 1944 he again had a series of upper respiratory infections. An inveterate smoker, he cut his daily quota of cigarettes from two packages to less than one. At about the same time, his increasing weariness overcame his pride and he discarded his heavy painful braces, giving up the pretense of walking. His last address to Congress was made sitting in a wheelchair.

His general decline continued, and in the pictures taken at Yalta in February 1945 Roosevelt looks haggard and worn; death seems to be written on his face. About March 1, 1945, full-time bodyguards were assigned to Vice President Harry Truman.

It has been reported that Roosevelt had a definite stroke in the latter part of March 1945 at Hyde Park. Dr. Rudolph Marx writes, "If this is true, it is difficult to understand why his physician permitted him to travel by train on March 30 to Warm Springs, or why he did not accompany him on the trip."[18] On the morning of April 12, 1945, at the "Little White House" in Georgia, Roosevelt was preparing a speech to be delivered over the radio in two days. Dr. McIntyre talked by phone with the doctor in charge of the president at Warm Springs and was assured that the patient was in excellent condition. During the noon hour the president sat in his leather chair while an artist made sketches for a new portrait. About one o'clock he suddenly looked up and said, "I have a terrific headache." He raised his left hand to his head, pressed it to his temple and ran it to his forehead—then slumped in his chair. He never regained consciousness and expired at 3:35 P.M. No autopsy was performed. "Massive cerebral hemorrhage" was given as the cause of death.

In the group of fifteen presidents holding office since 1900 (from Theodore Roosevelt through Ronald Reagan), those who have died have all succumbed from circulatory disorders (strokes or coronary thrombosis), with the exceptions of Presidents Hoover and Kennedy. Herbert Hoover died of cancer of the colon in 1964 at the age of 90,[22] and John Kennedy died in 1963 from an assassin's bullet to the brain.

Patricia Nixon

Pat Nixon arose shortly before 7:00 A.M. on the morning of July 7, 1976, and went to the kitchen to make coffee for her husband. She had trouble with her left hand when she tried to open a new can of coffee, and when the former president entered the room a few minutes later, he found her struggling with the top of the grapefruit juice bottle. He noticed immediately that the left corner of her mouth was drooping and that her speech was slightly slurred. He guessed then that she had had a stroke.

Julie Nixon relates these details in her book, *Pat Nixon: The Untold Story.*[23] The American public was particularly saddened and touched by the news of her illness because it occurred so promptly on the heels of the Watergate scandal, and many believed that Pat had been an innocent victim of that catastrophe. Richard Nixon publicly pinpointed the publication of *The Final Days* by Carl Bernstein and Bob Woodward as the precipitator of the stroke. Her physicians confirmed that stress could well have been a contributing factor. The book created a sensation, as the authors implied that President Nixon had been dangerously unbalanced and wrote that Mrs. Nixon "was becoming more and more reclusive and drinking heavily" and her marriage was loveless. Pat had been reading the book on the day before her stroke and also was in low spirits since the news of her husband's disbarment from the practice of law was to be released the next day by the New York State Bar.

Mrs. Nixon improved during the period following the stroke and by the sixth day was able to walk a few feet with aid from her husband. However, she faced long months of convalescence, rehabilitation exercises, and discouragement that was aggravated by depression. Stroke patients frequently experience dejection, and she was no exception. Three and a half months after the cerebral infarction, moving was still an effort and the clumsiness of her slight limp was debilitating and disheartening.

There has been little publicity of Mrs. Nixon's life in the past few years, and we do not know if she has sustained permanent neurologic deficits. Her daughter reports that she leads a restricted life and has been hospitalized four times in recent years because of pneumonia, bronchitis, and a second minor stroke in 1983.

References

1. Wepfer JJ: The History of the Sickness of Marcellus Malpighi, the Pope's Physician; with an Account of the Dissection of his Corps. From Baglivi, George: The Practice of Physick. London, Bell, p. 461, 1704 (English translation).

2. Major RH: Classic Descriptions of Disease. Springfield, IL, Charles C Thomas, pp. 515–516, 1939.

3. Mann J: Louis Pasteur: Founder of Bacteriology. New York, Charles Scribner's Sons, 1964.

4. L'Etang H: Lenin's final illness. Practitioner 204:587–590, 1970.

5. Payne R: The Life and Death of Lenin. New York, Simon and Schuster, 1964.

6. Friedlander WJ: About 3 old men—an inquiry into how cerebral arteriosclerosis has altered world politics. A neurologist's view. (Woodrow Wilson, Paul von Hindenberg, and Nikolai Lenin). Stroke 3:467–473, 1972.

7. Possony ST: Lenin: The Compulsive Revolutionary. London, George Allen & Unwin, 1966.

8. Payne R: The Rise and Fall of Stalin. New York, Avon Books, 1965.

9. Djilas M: Conversations with Stalin. New York, Harcourt, Brace & World, 1962.

10. Taylor B: Josef Stalin: A medical case history. Maryland State Med J 24(11):35–46, 1975.

11. Ulam AB: Stalin: The Man and His Era. New York, Viking Press, 1973.

12. Alliluyeva S: 20 Letters to a Friend. New York, Harper & Row, 1967.

13. Khrushchev NS: Khrushchev Remembers. Boston, Little, Brown & Co., 1970.

14. Taylor B: Victim of his fears. The Baltimore News American, May 4, 1975.

15. Bortoli G: The Death of Stalin. New York, Praeger, 1975.

16. Hingley R: Joseph Stalin: Man and Legend. New York, McGraw-Hill, 1974.

17. Eaton WJ: Gorbachev rips crimes by Stalin. Los Angeles Times as reported in the Houston Chronicle, November 3, 1987.

18. Marx R: The Health of the Presidents. New York, G. P. Putnam's Sons, 1960.

19. Robertson CW: Some observations on Presidential illnesses. Boston Med Quart 8, No. 2 and 3, June and September 1957.

20. Fishbein M: American presidents who had strokes. Postgrad Med 37:A200–208, March 1965.

21. Smith G: When the Cheering Stopped: The last years of Woodrow Wilson. New York, William Morrow, 1964.

22. Burner D: Herbert Hoover: A Public Life. New York, Alfred A. Knopf, 1979.

23. Eisenhower JN: Pat Nixon: The Untold Story. New York, Simon and Schuster, 1986.

SUBJECT INDEX

NAME INDEX